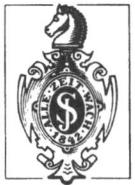

Fundamental Anatomy for Operative General Surgery is the first of a number of atlas-texts describing the essential anatomical basis of a range of common surgical procedures. Safe surgery is founded upon careful dissection and clear identification of vital structures. Knowledge of the appropriate anatomy and anatomical relations is therefore essential, not only during surgical training, but as the cornerstone of surgical practice. In this book clear line diagrams facing each page of text illustrate the important features that have to be identified. They highlight for trainees and practising surgeons features of the operations which are important anatomically, but do not attempt to give a complete description of the surgical procedure.

Other titles planned include:
- Orthopaedics
- Obstetrics and Gynaecology
- Cardiothoracic Surgery
- Plastic and Reconstructive Surgery
- Urology

S. J. Snooks and R. F. M. Wood

Fundamental Anatomy for Operative General Surgery

With 42 Figures

Springer-Verlag
London Berlin Heidelberg New York
Paris Tokyo

S. J. Snooks, MD, FRCS
Senior Surgical Registrar

R. F. M. Wood, MD, FRCS
Professor of Surgery

St. Bartholomew's Hospital
London EC1A 7BE, UK

ISBN-13:978-3-540-19535-1   e-ISBN-13:978-1-4471-1667-7
DOI: 10.1007/978-1-4471-1667-7

British Library Cataloguing in Publication Data
Snooks, S. J. (Steven James), 1953–
Fundamental anatomy for operative general surgery. 1. Man. Anatomy – For surgery
I. Title II. Wood, R. F. M. (Richard Frederick Marshall), 1943– .611'.00246171

Library of Congress Cataloging-in-Publication Data
Snooks, S. J. (Steven James)
Fundamental anatomy for operative general surgery.
Includes bibliographies and index.
1. Anatomy, Surgical and topographical. I. Wood, Richard F. M., 1943 . II.
Title. [DNLM: 1. Anatomy, Regional. 2. Surgery Operative. W0 101 W878f]
QM531.W65 1988   611   88–24840
ISBN-13:978-3-540-19535-1

Phototypeset by Tradeset Photosetting Ltd, Tewin Road, Welwyn Garden City, Herts.

2128/3916 – 543210 (Printed on acid-free paper)

Preface

Safe surgery is founded upon careful dissection and clear identification of vital structures. Knowledge of the appropriate anatomy and anatomical relations is therefore essential, not only during surgical training, but as the cornerstone of surgical practice.

The aim of this book is to describe the essential anatomical basis of a range of common procedures in general and vascular surgery. The large-format multi-volume texts on operative surgery, despite their undoubted excellence, are now too expensive for individual purchase. Single-volume books on operative surgery have been unable to devote sufficient attention to anatomical detail and the surgeon is left ploughing through anatomy texts, often failing to find illustrations which demonstrate clearly the features that are important in an operative dissection. The present text highlights features of the operations which are important anatomically while not attempting to give a complete description of the operative procedure. A combination of line diagrams and cross sections has been used to provide the topographical detail.

The volume is aimed mainly at surgeons in training, to help them on a day-to-day basis and to provide a text which will be useful in revising for post-graduate examinations in surgery. It is also hoped that the book will be of use to practising surgeons, providing an easy means of highlighting important anatomical aspects of the procedures they perform relatively infrequently.

1989   S.J.S.
R.F.M.W.

Contents

I. Head and Neck

Superficial Parotidectomy

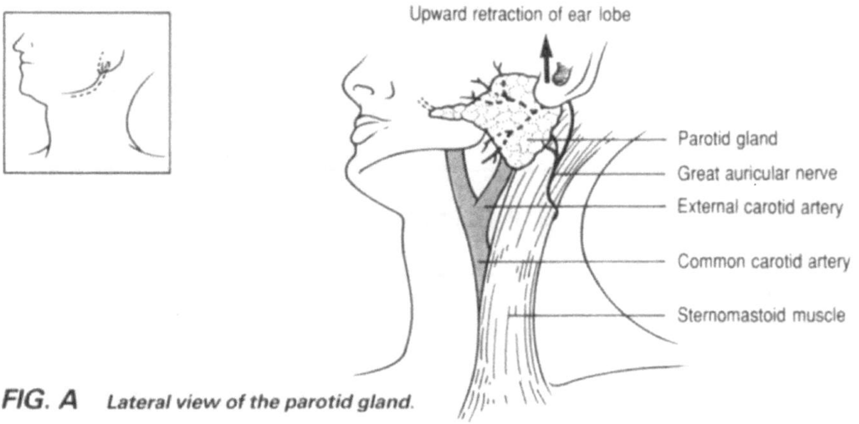

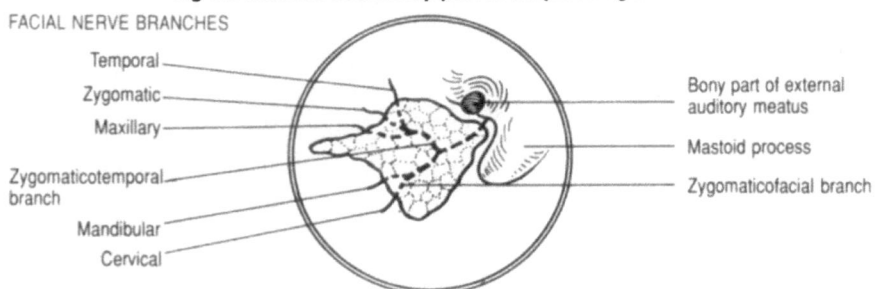

Upward retraction of ear lobe

Parotid gland
Great auricular nerve
External carotid artery
Common carotid artery
Sternomastoid muscle

FIG. A *Lateral view of the parotid gland.*

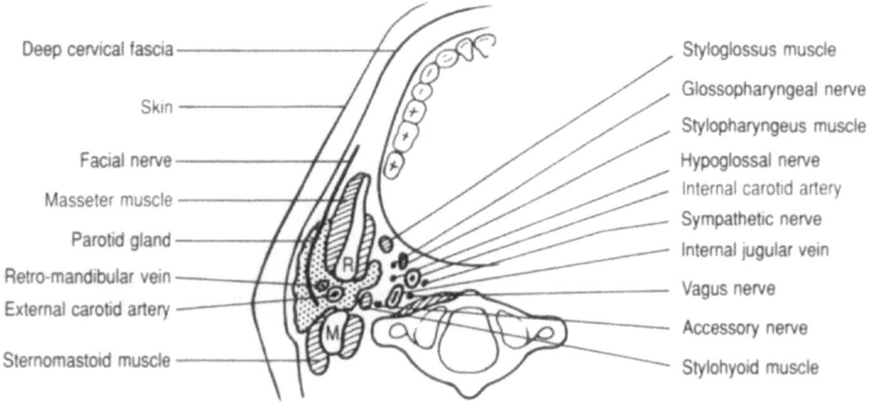

Deep cervical fascia
Skin
Facial nerve
Masseter muscle
Parotid gland
Retro-mandibular vein
External carotid artery
Sternomastoid muscle

Styloglossus muscle
Glossopharyngeal nerve
Stylopharyngeus muscle
Hypoglossal nerve
Internal carotid artery
Sympathetic nerve
Internal jugular vein
Vagus nerve
Accessory nerve
Stylohyoid muscle

FIG. B *Transverse section through the ramus (R) of the mandible and the mastoid process (M) demonstrating the relations of the deep part of the parotid gland.*

FACIAL NERVE BRANCHES
Temporal
Zygomatic
Maxillary
Zygomaticotemporal branch
Mandibular
Cervical

Bony part of external auditory meatus
Mastoid process
Zygomaticofacial branch

FIG. C *Lateral view of facial nerve leaving the skull and dividing.*

2

The serous secreting parotid gland extends from the zygomatic arch to just below the angle of the jaw (fig. a). The facial nerve separates the superficial portion of the gland, lying on the masseter muscle, from the deep component, which penetrates into the space between the ramus of the mandible and the mastoid process (fig. b). Most pathological processes involve the superficial portion of the gland and parotidectomy can be achieved with complete preservation of the facial nerve and its terminal branches. There are two or three lymph nodes on the surface of the gland or embedded in its substance. These nodes drain the anterior part of the scalp and the face above the level of the mouth.

- The incision should be designed so that it does not leave a pointed skin flap behind the ear, because of the risk of devascularisation. It should not be placed too close to the lower border of the mandible in order to avoid damage to the mandibular branch of the facial nerve.

- The anterior skin flap should not be raised beyond the anterior border of the gland, so as to preserve the anterior branches of the facial nerve (fig. a).

- Posteriorly the external jugular vein and great auricular nerve (fig. a) are identified and may have to be divided to achieve adequate mobilisation of the lower pole of the gland.

- The facial nerve leaves the skull via the stylomastoid foramen at the apex of the inverted "v" sulcus between the mastoid process and the bony part of the external auditory meatus (fig. c). The nerve should be traced down into the gland to find the correct plane of dissection.

- To avoid damage to the branches of the facial nerve the partially mobilised gland should be repeatedly reorientated with all the facial nerve branches in their correct position before dissection proceeds anteriorly.

Excision of Submandibular Gland

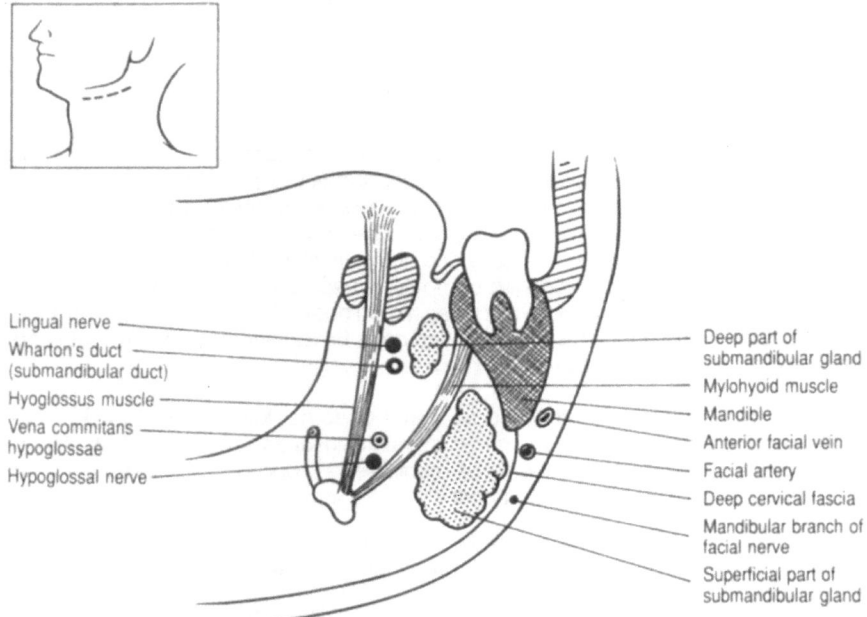

FIG. A *Right sided coronal section through the body of the mandible.*

Lingual nerve
Wharton's duct (submandibular duct)
Hyoglossus muscle
Vena commitans hypoglossae
Hypoglossal nerve

Deep part of submandibular gland
Mylohyoid muscle
Mandible
Anterior facial vein
Facial artery
Deep cervical fascia
Mandibular branch of facial nerve
Superficial part of submandibular gland

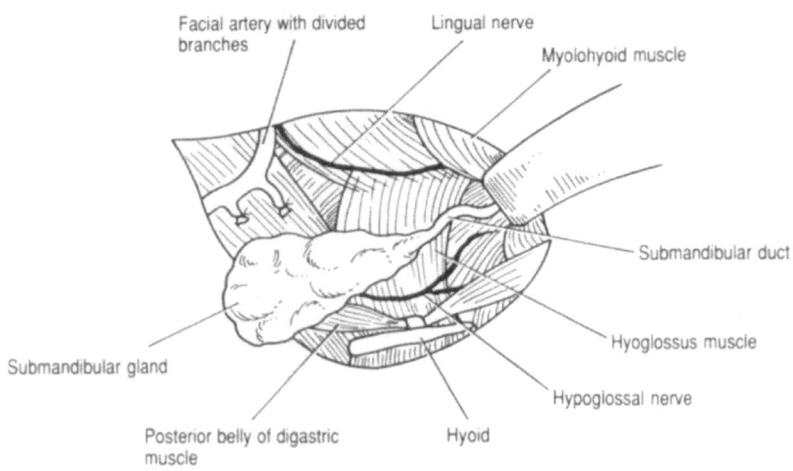

Facial artery with divided branches
Lingual nerve
Myolohyoid muscle
Submandibular duct
Hyoglossus muscle
Hypoglossal nerve
Hyoid
Posterior belly of digastric muscle
Submandibular gland

FIG. B *Deep relations of the submandibular gland. Lateral view of the dissection.*

Excision of Submandibular Gland

The submandibular gland is a serous secreting salivary gland situated between the mandible, the medial pterygoid muscle laterally, and the mylohyoid and hyoglossus muscles medially.

- The incision to remove the gland should be placed approximately 2 cm beneath and parallel to the lower border of the mandible to avoid trauma to the mandibular division of the facial nerve (fig. a).

- The facial artery, which often has to be divided with the anterior facial vein (figs. a and b), also lies superficial to the deep cervical fascia.

- The anterior portion of the gland is dissected off the mylohyoid muscle.

- The facial artery is close to the posterior portion of the gland and is often tethered to it by two branches which supply the gland substance (fig. b).

- The posterior border of the mylohyoid muscle is retracted anteriorly to expose the deep part of the gland (fig. b).

- Medial to the deep part of the gland lie the lingual and hypoglossal nerves. The lingual nerve is closely related to the deep part of the gland and duct. Care must be taken to avoid damage to the lingual nerve when the submandibular duct is clamped and divided as far anteriorly as possible (fig. a).

Cervical Sympathectomy

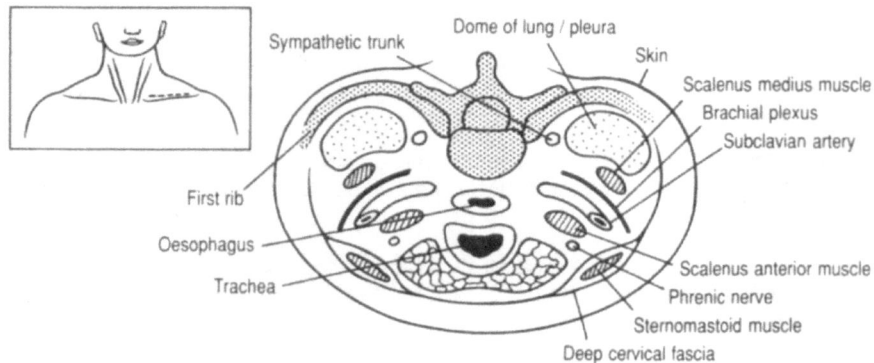

FIG. A *Transverse section through the root of the neck.*

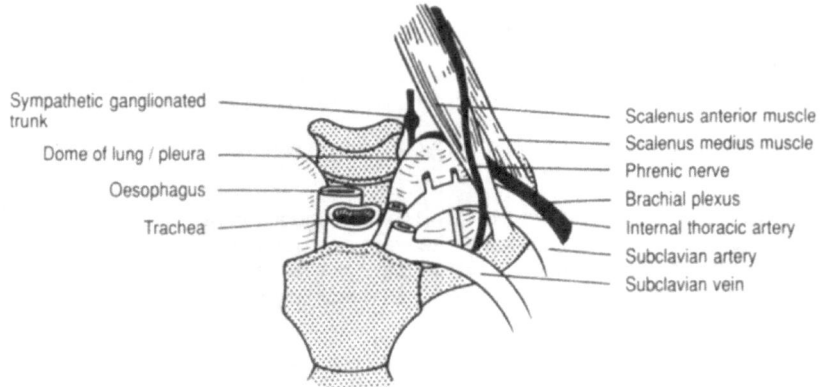

FIG. B *Anteroposterior view of the root of the neck.*

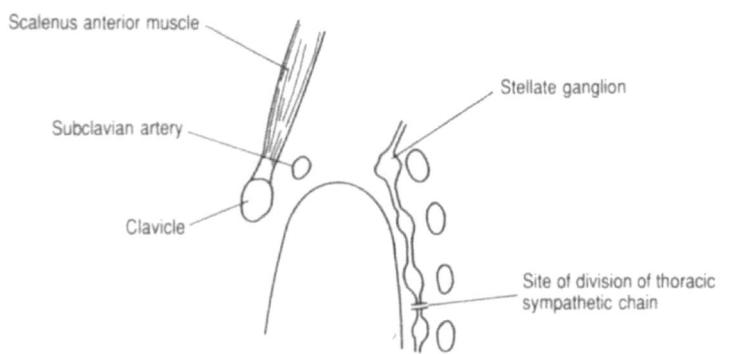

FIG. C *Anatomical position of the cervical and thoracic sympathetic ganglia (lateral view).*

Sympathetic innervation to the upper limbs is from the white rami communicantes (T5–T9) which relay in the inferior and middle cervical ganglia and travel with the roots of the brachial plexus (C5, C6: middle) and (C7, C8: stellate or inferior).

Anterior supraclavicular approach:

- The external jugular vein and the inferior belly of the omohyoid muscle are divided to gain access to the deep structures. The posterior triangle of the neck is entered by retracting the sternomastoid muscle medially (fig. a).

- In left sided operations damage to the thoracic duct must be avoided. This crosses everything in the neck except the carotid sheath.

- The scalenus anterior muscle which lies on the floor of the posterior triangle of the neck (fig. b) is divided, separating and preserving the phrenic nerve which descends along its anterior surface (fig. b).

- The subclavian artery lies behind the scalenus anterior muscle and anterior to the brachial plexus and scalenus medius muscle (fig. b).

- In order to reach the cervical sympathetic chain the dome of the pleura lying behind scalenus medius is depressed (fig. b), avoiding tears which would cause a pneumothorax.

- The sympathetic ganglionated trunk is the only structure running vertically (fig. c) behind the dome of the lung.

- The sympathetic chain is divided just beneath the third thoracic ganglion (fig. c). If the stellate ganglion is not dissected out Horner's syndrome should not occur.

Thyroidectomy

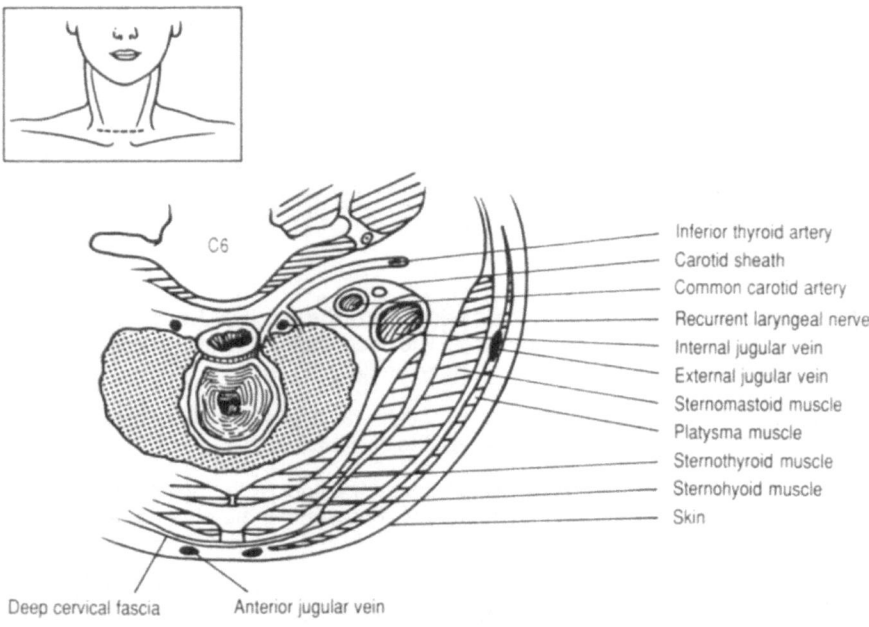

FIG. A *Transverse section through the neck (C6).*

Labels (Fig. A):
- C6
- Inferior thyroid artery
- Carotid sheath
- Common carotid artery
- Recurrent laryngeal nerve
- Internal jugular vein
- External jugular vein
- Sternomastoid muscle
- Platysma muscle
- Sternothyroid muscle
- Sternohyoid muscle
- Skin
- Deep cervical fascia
- Anterior jugular vein

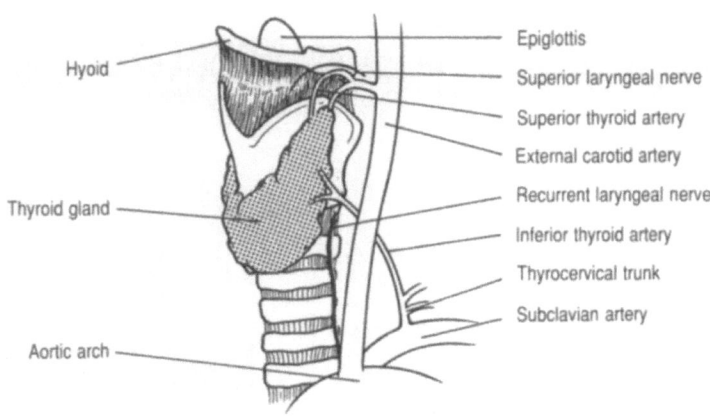

FIG. B *Lateral view of the thyroid gland and larynx.*

Labels (Fig. B):
- Hyoid
- Thyroid gland
- Aortic arch
- Epiglottis
- Superior laryngeal nerve
- Superior thyroid artery
- External carotid artery
- Recurrent laryngeal nerve
- Inferior thyroid artery
- Thyrocervical trunk
- Subclavian artery

The thyroid gland is approached via a transverse cervical incision midway between the thyroid notch and the sternal notch. The incision is often made too low, in the mistaken belief that it will be more cosmetic. Unfortunately, this results in the need for a much longer scar to achieve sufficient mobilisation of the upper skin flap.

- The anterior jugular veins, and their communicating branch in the space of Burns, can easily be traumatised when deepening the incision (fig. a).

- The midline can be easily identified. The midline lies on either side of the two groups of strap muscles: sternohyoid (most superficial), thyrohyoid (above) and the underlying sternothyroid, applied to the surface of the gland (fig. a).

- The key to effective thyroid surgery is identification of the vascular connections of the gland. The middle and inferior thyroid veins are identified first.

- The tributaries forming the middle thyroid vein are easily seen on the surface of the gland and the vein should be divided early to allow the thyroid lobe to be dislocated forward. The inferior thyroid vein running from the lower pole can be divided close to the gland without risk to deeper structures, i.e. the recurrent laryngeal nerve (fig. a).

- The superior pole of the thyroid gland can only be mobilised after dividing the superior thyroid vessels. The superior thyroid artery (branch of the external carotid artery) and the superior thyroid vein are in a perivascular sheath at the apex of the upper pole (fig. b). The superior laryngeal nerve runs with superior thyroid vessels before piercing the thyrohyoid membrane (fig. b).

- The inferior thyroid artery (branch of the thyrocervical trunk) emerges from beneath the carotid artery (figs. a and b). Its terminal branches surround the recurrent laryngeal nerve. Consequently it is best to retract the common carotid artery and ligate the inferior thyroid artery in continuity as far laterally as possible.

- Preserving the recurrent laryngeal nerve is of paramount importance in thyroid surgery. Therefore, the nerve should always be visualised. On drawing the thyroid lobe forward it can be seen below the level of the inferior thyroid artery as a white structure running vertically in the tracheo-oesophageal groove. The tiny nutrient artery on the surface of the nerve is a useful aid to positive identification.

Thyroglossal Cyst

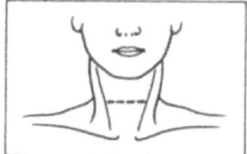

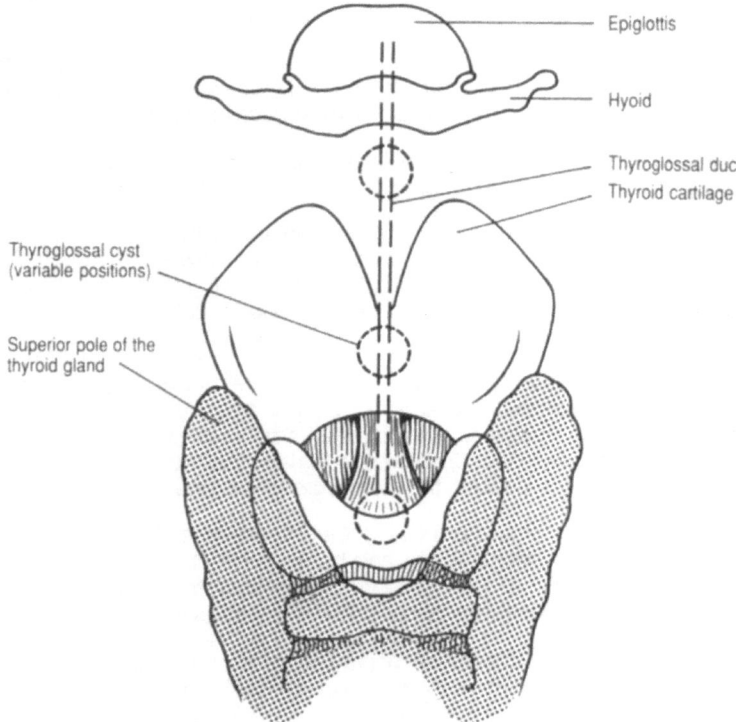

Epiglottis

Hyoid

Thyroglossal duct
Thyroid cartilage

Thyroglossal cyst
(variable positions)

Superior pole of the
thyroid gland

FIG. A *Anterior view of the thyroid and cricoid cartilages and hyoid bone.*

Thyroglossal Cyst

The thyroglossal duct develops embryologically from the first pharyngeal pouch and arches behind the hyoid bone. Having descended into the neck it divides into the lateral lobes and the isthmus of the thyroid gland. Failure of normal obliteration of the duct may allow the formation of a thyroglossal cyst. In addition remnants of thyroid tissue may be present in the line of the duct from the foramen caecum of the tongue (the lingual thyroid) to the pyramidal lobe at the thyroid isthmus. A thyroglossal cyst is usually present in the midline of the neck above the isthmus of the thyroid gland and usually moves upwards on protrusion of the tongue.

- Care must be taken to remove the cyst in continuity with any ductal remnant. The cyst and attached remnant should be turned upwards and a segment of the hyoid excised in the midline so that the duct can be traced up to the floor of the mouth (fig. a).

Tracheostomy

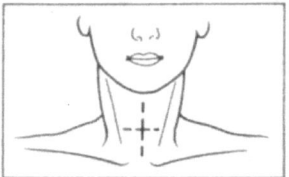

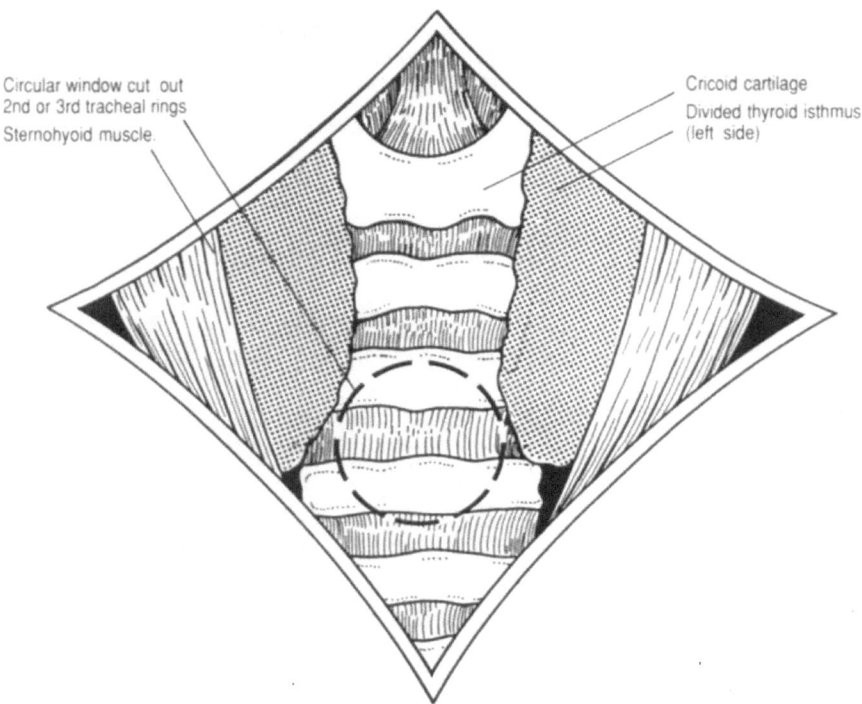

Circular window cut out
2nd or 3rd tracheal rings

Sternohyoid muscle.

Cricoid cartilage

Divided thyroid isthmus
(left side)

FIG. A *Anterior view of the trachea after division of the thyroid isthmus.*

Elective tracheostomy is performed via a transverse cervical incision as for thyroidectomy. Emergency tracheostomy may be performed via a longitudinal midline incision.

- The thyroid isthmus is divided in the midline (fig. a).

- A 1-cm diameter tracheal window is cut beneath the first tracheal ring so as to avoid tracheal stenosis (fig. a).

OR

- An inverted u-shaped incision is made below the first tracheal ring. Suture of the apex of the "U" to the lower skin flap aids safe placement and replacement of the tracheostomy tube.

Pharyngeal Pouch

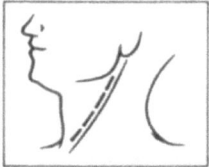

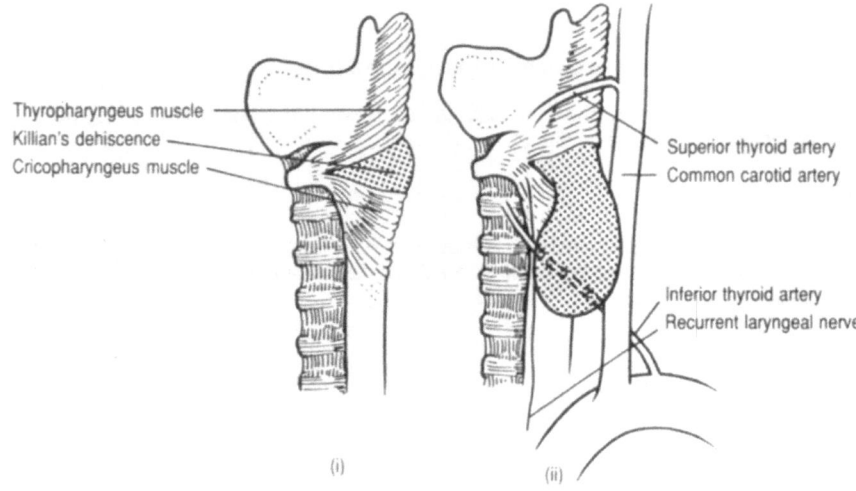

Thyropharyngeus muscle
Killian's dehiscence
Cricopharyngeus muscle

Superior thyroid artery
Common carotid artery

Inferior thyroid artery
Recurrent laryngeal nerve

(i)

(ii)

FIG. A *Lateral view of the laryngopharynx with (i)
and without (ii) a pharyngeal pouch.*

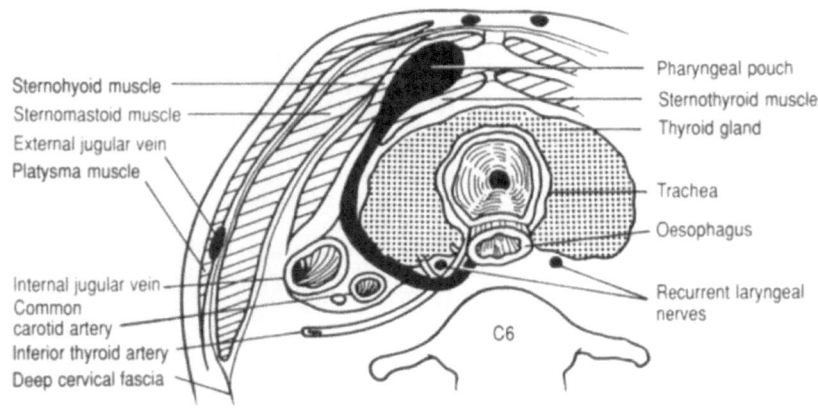

Sternohyoid muscle
Sternomastoid muscle
External jugular vein
Platysma muscle

Pharyngeal pouch
Sternothyroid muscle
Thyroid gland

Trachea

Oesophagus

Internal jugular vein
Common
carotid artery
Inferior thyroid artery
Deep cervical fascia

C6

Recurrent laryngeal
nerves

FIG. B *Left sided transverse section through the
neck (C6).*

Pharyngeal Pouch

The pharyngeal pouch is a protrusion through Killian's dehiscence. This is a weak area of the posterior pharyngeal wall between the thyropharyngeus and the cricopharyngeus muscles, which are both components of the inferior constrictor muscle (fig. a). Usually the pouch protrudes to the left.

- An oblique incision along the anterior border of sternomastoid offers good exposure of the lateral part of the thyroid gland and carotid sheath. The muscle is retracted laterally.

- Mobilisation of the thyroid gland is often required (fig. a), with division of the middle thyroid vein and inferior thyroid artery (p. 8).

- The carotid sheath is retracted posteriorly in order to reach the neck of the pharyngeal pouch (fig. b).

- The neck of the sac should be closed to prevent narrowing of the pharynx. In addition a vertical cricopharyngeal myotomy is usually performed, dividing the hypertrophied circular muscle.

Branchial Cyst and Fistula

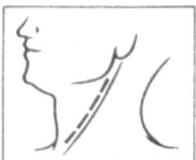

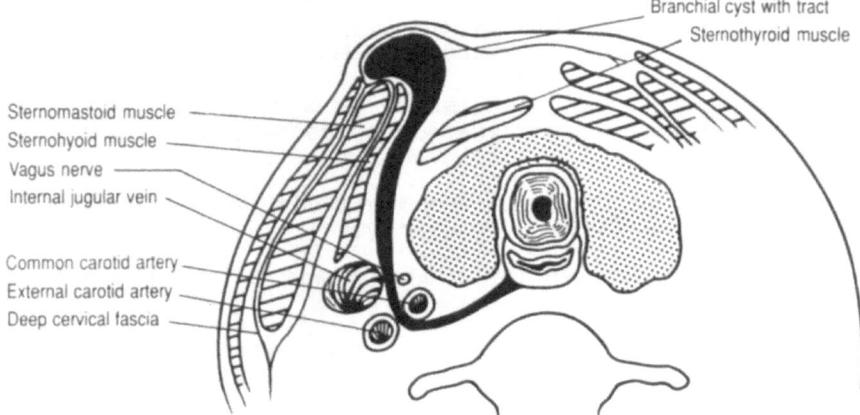

Branchial cyst with tract
Sternothyroid muscle

Sternomastoid muscle
Sternohyoid muscle
Vagus nerve
Internal jugular vein

Common carotid artery
External carotid artery
Deep cervical fascia

FIG. A *Transverse section through the neck (C6).*

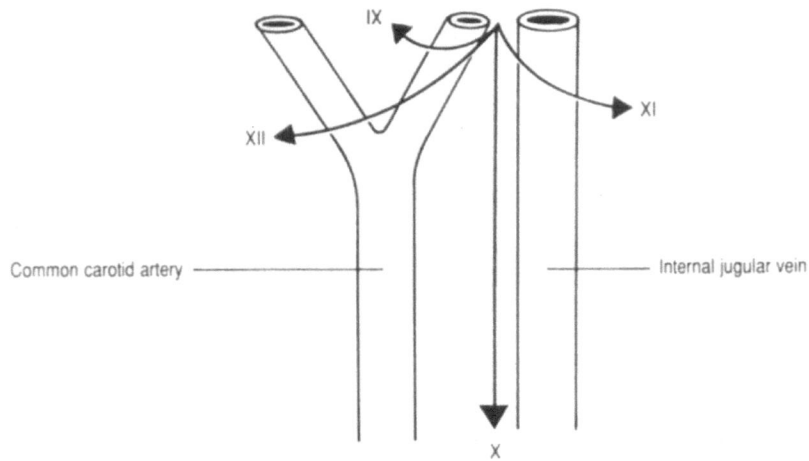

IX

XI

XII

Common carotid artery

Internal jugular vein

X

FIG. B *Lateral view of the vessels at the base of the skull and their relationship to the cranial nerves IX, X, XI and XII.*

Branchial Cyst and Fistula

A branchial cyst forms from the vestigial remnants of the second branchial cleft and protrudes along the anterior border of the upper third of the sternomastoid muscle. Occasionally the cyst is associated with a track which is attached to the pharynx as in a branchial fistula (fig. a). A branchial fistula most probably represents a persistent second branchial cleft. The external orifice of the fistula is situated in the lower third of the neck near the anterior border of the sternomastoid muscle. The internal orifice is located on the posterior pillar of the fauces behind the tonsil; alternatively the fistula may end blindly on the lateral pharyngeal wall.

- The same incision along the anterior border of sternomastoid can be used as for excising a pharyngeal pouch.

- The fistula or track is followed and usually passes between the internal and external carotid arteries (fig. a), where it passes deep to the posterior belly of the digastric muscle and superficial to the hypoglossal, glossopharyngeal and spinal accessory nerves (fig. b).

II. Abdomen

Truncal Vagotomy with Pyloroplasty and Highly Selective Vagotomy

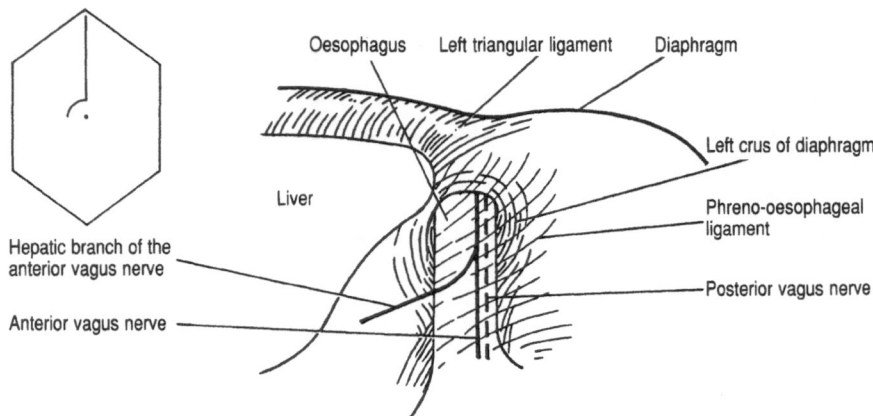

Oesophagus Left triangular ligament Diaphragm

Left crus of diaphragm

Liver

Phreno-oesophageal ligament

Hepatic branch of the anterior vagus nerve

Posterior vagus nerve

Anterior vagus nerve

FIG. A *Relations of the intra-abdominal oesophagus.*

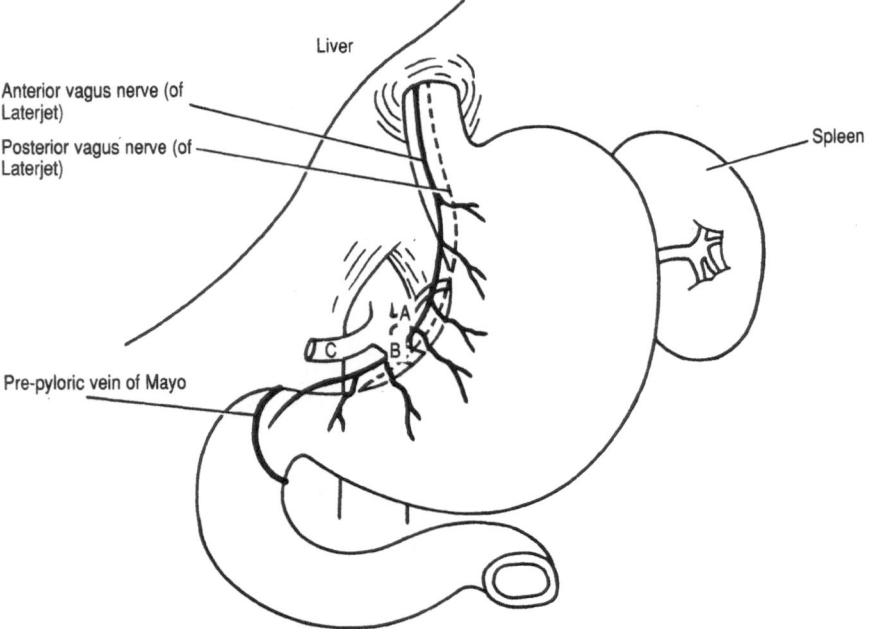

Liver

Anterior vagus nerve (of Laterjet)

Posterior vagus nerve (of Laterjet)

Spleen

Pre-pyloric vein of Mayo

FIG. B *Relations of the stomach to the anterior and posterior nerves of Laterjet and branches of the coeliac axis (A, left gastric artery; B, splenic artery; C, common hepatic artery).*

Truncal Vagotomy with Pyloroplasty and Highly Selective Vagotomy

The operation is usually performed via an upper midline incision, retracting the xiphisternum forwards to visualise the oesophageal hiatus.

- Mobilisation of the intra-abdominal part of the oesophagus is achieved by division of the left hepatic triangular ligament (fig. a) and the phreno-oesophageal ligament together with the peritoneum overlying the oesophagus (fig. a). The anterior vagus nerve is closely applied to the anterior surface of the oesophagus. It can be felt with the tip of the index finger as a string-like structure when the oesophagus is put under tension. The posterior vagus nerve is usually separate from the oesophagus. It can be picked up by passing a finger behind the oesophagus from left to right and is more chord-like in nature (fig. a).

- Truncal vagotomy requires the addition of a drainage procedure, either a pyloroplasty or a gastro-enterostomy. The site of the pylorus is identified by locating the pre-pyloric vein of Mayo (fig. b). In a Heineke–Mikulicz pyloroplasty a 5-cm longitudinal incision is positioned centrally over the pylorus and closed transversely.

- Highly selective vagotomy (parietal cell vagotomy) preserves the innervation of the pylorus and does not require the addition of a drainage procedure. The nerves of Laterjet, the continuation of the anterior and posterior vagal trunks along the lesser curve of the stomach, are identified (fig. b). The main vagal trunks are carefully preserved but branches to the oesophagus and cardia are divided. The body of the stomach is innervated by small branches of the nerves of Laterjet which run alongside the vessels to the lesser curve. Division of the vascular connections achieves denervation of the body of the stomach (fig. b). The nerve supply to the pyloric antrum is preserved to allow normal gastric emptying.

Total Gastrectomy

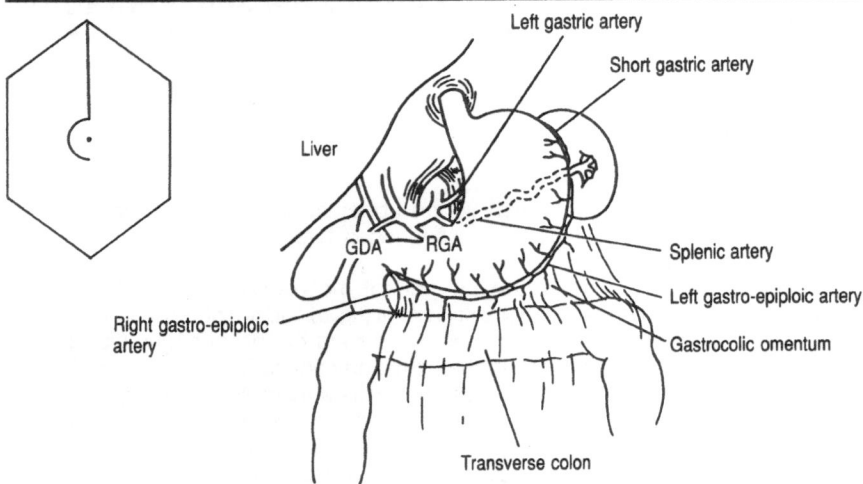

FIG. A *Blood supply to the stomach. GDA, gastroduodenal artery; RGA, right gastric artery.*

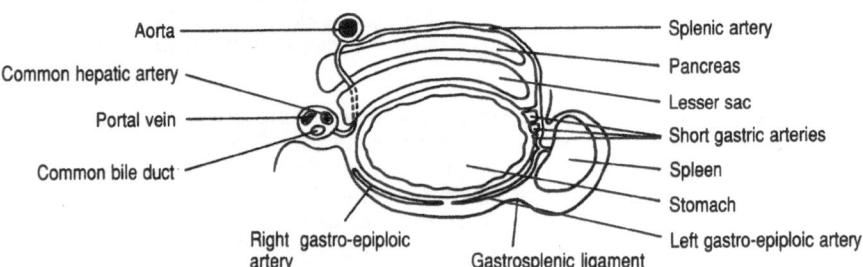

FIG. B *Transverse section through stomach and free edge of lesser omentum depicting the lesser sac.*

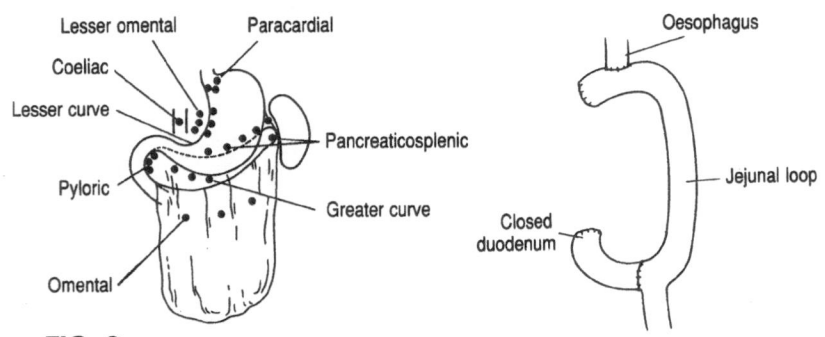

FIG. C *Main lymphatic drainage of the stomach/groups of lymph nodes.*

FIG. D *Roux-en-Y reconstruction.*

Total Gastrectomy

The main indication for total gastrectromy is carcinoma of the stomach. In attempting a curative resection the stomach may be removed en bloc with the spleen, the greater omentum and the lymph nodes in the lesser omentum.

- The greater omentum is separated from the transverse colon and the lesser sac entered by division of the gastrocolic omentum (fig. a). This enables both mobilisation of the greater curve of the stomach and inspection of the posterior gastric wall to assess tumour penetration through the lesser sac into the pancreas and/or posterior abdominal wall.

- If the spleen is to be removed with the specimen it should be mobilised and the splenic artery and vein divided at the tail of the pancreas, preserving the short gastric vessels. If the spleen is to be retained the short gastric vessels should be divided in the gastrosplenic ligament (fig. b), thus freeing the greater curve of the stomach.

- The origin of the left gastric artery, arising from the coeliac axis, should be identified (fig. a). Division of the vessel at this level allows the lesser omentum and its lymph nodes to be dissected in continuity with the stomach (fig. c).

- The right gastric artery (fig. a) is a branch of the common hepatic artery (figs. a and b) and arises where the hepatic artery enters the lesser omentum. The right gastric artery supplies the stomach and the superior part of the duodenum. It is divided when mobilising the lower part of the stomach and the first part of the duodenum. This allows the lesser omentum to be divided preserving the common bile duct, common hepatic artery and portal vein which lie in its free edge (fig. b).

- Reconstruction can be achieved using a Roux-en-Y loop (fig. d).

- If the greater omentum is to be removed it has to be dissected off the transverse colon and removed with the stomach. The transverse mesocolon may be adherent to the greater omentum thereby endangering the middle colic vessels and consequently the integrity of colonic blood supply.

Partial Gastrectomy

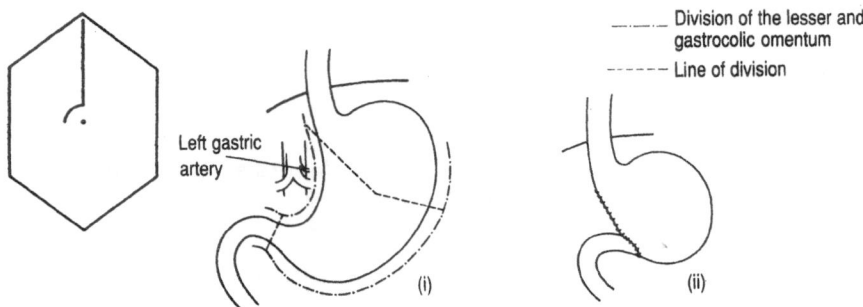

Left gastric artery

.... Division of the lesser and gastrocolic omentum

------- Line of division

(i)

(ii)

FIG. A *Billroth I gastrectomy showing the division of the lesser and gastrocolic omentum and the line of division.*

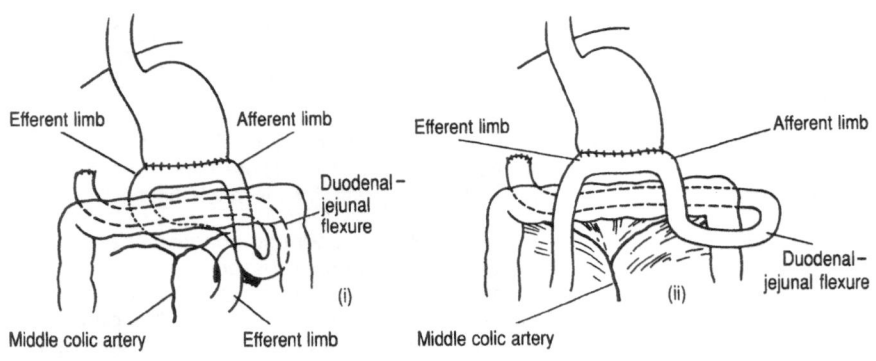

Efferent limb

Afferent limb

Duodenal - jejunal flexure

Middle colic artery

Efferent limb

(i)

Efferent limb

Afferent limb

Duodenal - jejunal flexure

Middle colic artery

(ii)

FIG. B *Retro-colic (i) and ante-colic (ii) gastro-jejunostomy reconstructions as in a Polya gastrectomy.*

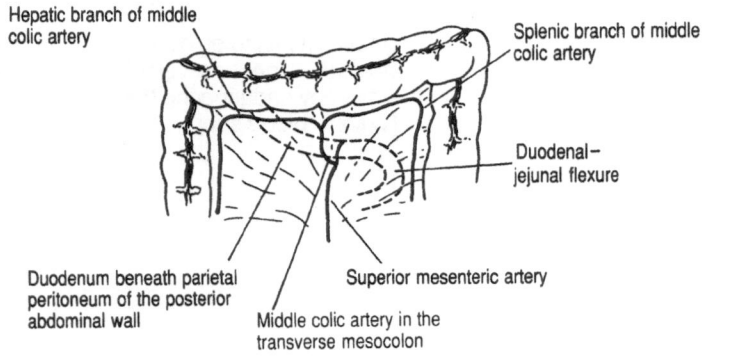

Hepatic branch of middle colic artery

Splenic branch of middle colic artery

Duodenal - jejunal flexure

Duodenum beneath parietal peritoneum of the posterior abdominal wall

Middle colic artery in the transverse mesocolon

Superior mesenteric artery

FIG. C *The transverse mesocolon and its vessels.*

The Billroth I gastrectomy, restoring continuity with the duodenum, was originally described as a treatment for duodenal ulceration. The procedure is now employed for lesions of the distal third of the stomach and is performed relatively rarely. Polya gastrectomy, with oversewing of the duodenal stump and the formation of a gastro-enterostomy, is used to achieve a more extensive gastric resection.

Billroth I

- If the procedure is being performed for a benign lesion the vessels along the greater and lesser curves can be divided close to the stomach.

- To achieve sufficient mobilisation of the stomach for an anastomosis that will not be under tension it is usually necessary to divide the left gastric artery at its origin from the coeliac axis (fig. a).

Polya

- Reconstruction of the gastrointestinal tract can be achieved by either a retro-colic or an ante-colic gastro-jejunostomy (fig. b).

- In performing a retro-colic anastomosis the transverse colon should first be held up anteriorly to display the branches of the middle colic artery (fig. c). An appropriate opening can then be made in the transverse mesocolon to enable the retro-colic anastomosis to be performed (figs. b and c).

Ivor Lewis Approach to the Intrathoracic Oesophagus

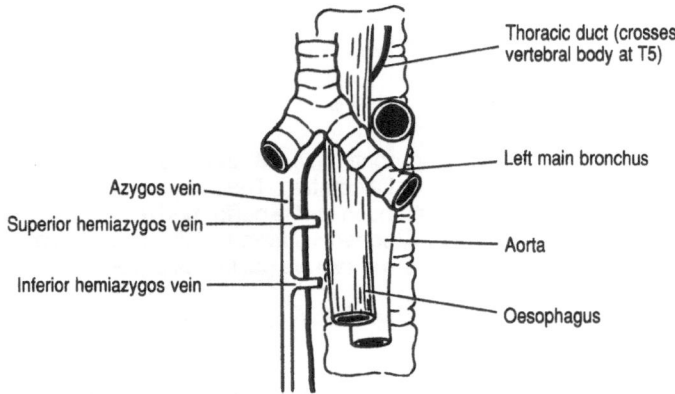

FIG. A *Anterior aspect of the posterior mediastinum.*

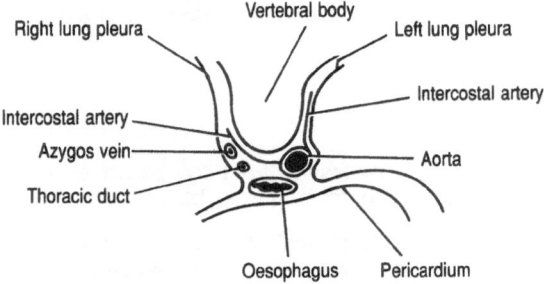

FIG. B *Transverse section through the mediastinum.*

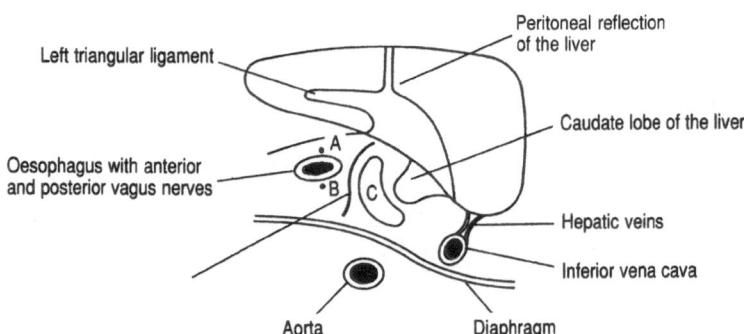

FIG. C *Transverse section through the upper abdomen. A and B, anterior and posterior vagus nerves; C, upper recess of the lesser sac.*

Ivor Lewis Approach to the Intrathoracic Oesophagus

Carcinomas of the lower oesophagus can be treated by the Ivor Lewis procedure. The initial step is to mobilise the stomach as in a total gastrectomy (p. 22). The oesophagus is approached through a right thoracotomy incision and the tumour excised. The gastric remnant is drawn into the chest and anastomosed to the divided end of the oesophagus. The proximal extent of the dissection from the right side of the chest is limited by the aortic arch which crosses the oesophagus at the level of T4.

- The thoracic duct and azygos vein lie behind and to the right of the oesophagus in the posterior mediastinum (figs. a and b).

- The thoracic aorta is medial to the oesophagus and gives off segmental intercostal arteries. These, in turn, have small branches which supply the oesophagus (fig. b). Preservation of an adequate oesophageal blood supply is one of the key factors in achieving primary healing of the anastomosis. Unnecessarily extensive mobilisation of the oesophagus should therefore be avoided.

- Within the abdomen the left lobe of the liver overlies the oesophagogastric junction. The left gastric artery runs upwards in the lesser omentum to supply the lower end of the oesophagus. The upper recess of the lesser sac lies to the right of the oesophagus (fig. c).

Cholecystectomy and the Biliary Tree

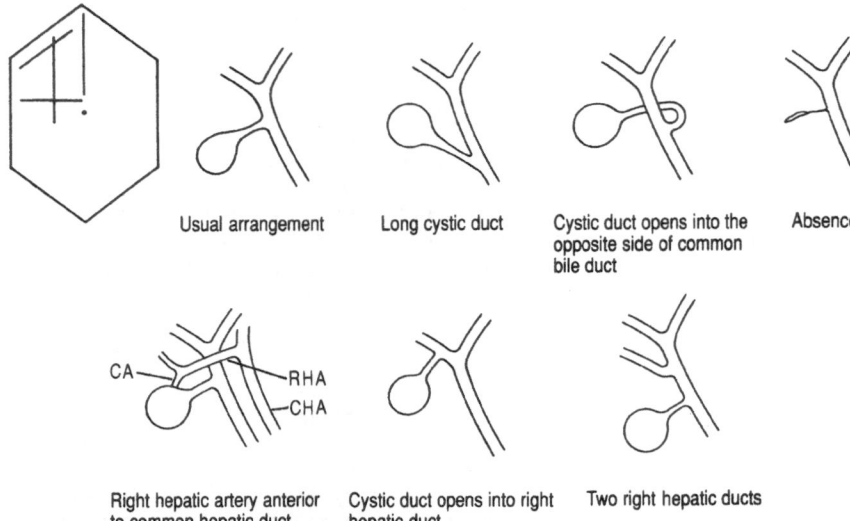

Usual arrangement   Long cystic duct   Cystic duct opens into the opposite side of common bile duct   Absence

Right hepatic artery anterior to common hepatic duct   Cystic duct opens into right hepatic duct   Two right hepatic ducts

FIG. A *Variations of the biliary tree and its vasculature. NB: The right hepatic artery (RHA) may be a branch of the superior mesenteric artery. CA, cystic artery; CHA, common hepatic artery.*

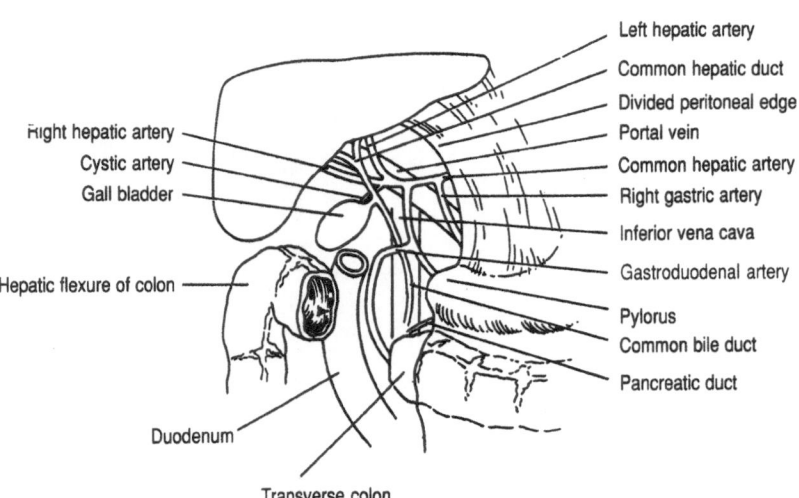

Right hepatic artery
Cystic artery
Gall bladder

Hepatic flexure of colon

Duodenum

Transverse colon

Left hepatic artery
Common hepatic duct
Divided peritoneal edge
Portal vein
Common hepatic artery
Right gastric artery
Inferior vena cava
Gastroduodenal artery
Pylorus
Common bile duct
Pancreatic duct

FIG. B *Relations of the gall bladder and biliary ducts.*

Cholecystectomy and the Biliary Tree

There is considerable variability in the anatomy of the biliary tree. This applies, in particular, to the cystic duct and its junction with the common hepatic duct, and the biliary tree's relationship to cystic and hepatic arteries (fig. a).

• Before the cystic duct is divided in the course of performing a cholecystectomy the junction between the cystic and common hepatic ducts should be demonstrated, i.e. the "T" junction (fig. b). Confirmation of the anatomy can be achieved by operative cholangiography. If the junction of the cystic duct and common hepatic duct is difficult to dissect it is safer, in order to avoid damage to the biliary tree, to free the fundus of the gall bladder from the liver and work carefully towards the porta hepatis (fundus first or retrograde cholecystectomy).

• The cystic artery usually passes underneath the common hepatic duct, but may cross above, where it can be confused with the right hepatic artery (figs. a and b).

• Often a fold of peritoneum has to be divided adjacent to the common hepatic duct in order to identify the cystic artery (fig. b).

• The common bile duct is approximately 5 mm in diameter in the absence of extrahepatic biliary obstruction. It varies in length from 5 cm to 12 cm depending upon the length of the common hepatic duct.

• The first part of the common bile duct lies in the free border of the lesser omentum forming the anterior boundary of the epiploic foramen, with the hepatic artery to the left and the portal vein posteriorly (fig. b).

• The second part of the common bile duct passes posterior to the duodenum with the gastroduodenal artery situated to the left. As the duct passes inferiorly it curves to the right and is embedded in the head of the pancreas, which separates it from the inferior vena cava (fig. b).

• The common bile duct is supplied by a fine network of vessels which in the main run longitudinally. The duct should therefore only be incised longitudinally, and to prevent stricture formation diathermy is best avoided.

• The common bile duct and pancreatic duct usually unite to form the ampulla of Vater with a common opening into the duodenum. However, the ducts may open separately into the second part of the duodenum and it is important to be aware of this potential anomaly when undertaking a transduodenal sphincterotomy procedure.

The Subphrenic Spaces

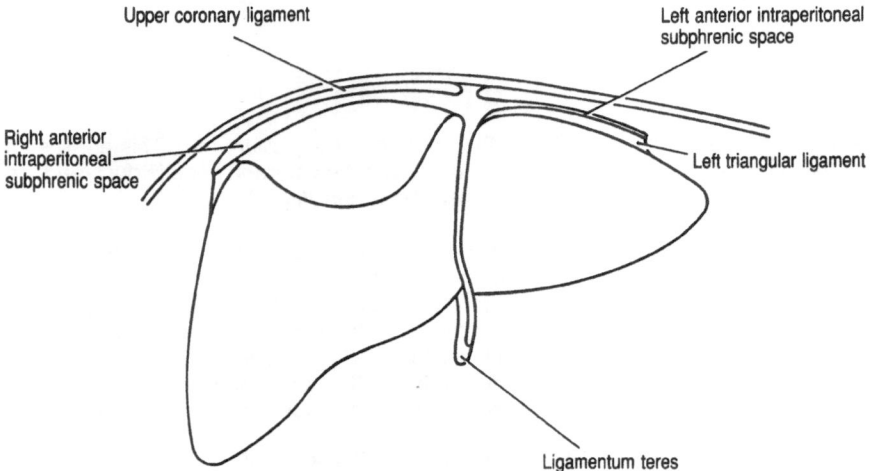

Upper coronary ligament

Left anterior intraperitoneal subphrenic space

Right anterior intraperitoneal subphrenic space

Left triangular ligament

Ligamentum teres

FIG. A *The anterior subphrenic spaces.*

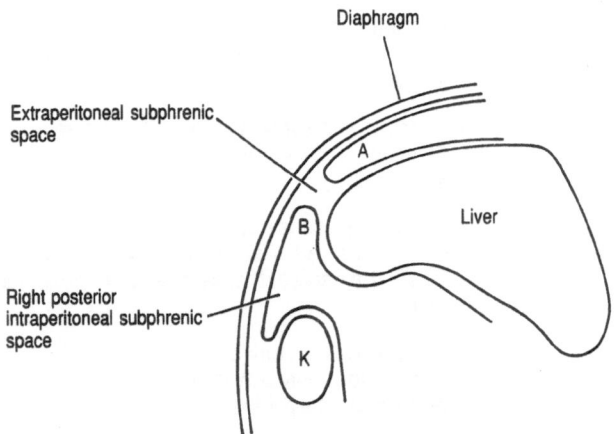

Diaphragm

Extraperitoneal subphrenic space

Right posterior intraperitoneal subphrenic space

Liver

A

B

K

FIG. B *The posterior (right) and extraperitoneal subphrenic spaces (sagittal section). A, upper coronary ligament; B, lower coronary ligament; K, kidney.*

The Subphrenic spaces are "potential spaces" below the diaphragm produced by the peritoneal folds around the liver (figs. a, b and c). The spaces are all intraperitoneal with the exception of the small extraperitoneal compartment between the diaphragm and the bare area of the liver (figs. b and c).

Right Anterior Subphrenic Space (fig. a)

- Superiorly this space is bounded by the upper coronary ligament and inferiorly by the general peritoneal cavity (fig. a).

- The anterior and lateral margins are the diaphragm and anterior abdominal wall. The right lobe of the liver forms the posterior boundary of the space and the medial extent is limited by the falciform ligament.

- The right anterior space is continuous with the right posterior space, allowing infection to spread from one space to the other.

Left Anterior Subphrenic Space (fig. a)

- Superiorly this space is bounded by the left triangular ligament and inferiorly by the general peritoneal cavity (fig. a).

- The falciform ligament forms the medial border and the space extends laterally as far as the spleen.

- Anteroposteriorly the space extends from the abdominal wall and diaphragm to the left lobe of the liver.

Right Posterior Subphrenic Space: Pouch of Rutherford-Morrison (fig. b)

- Superiorly this space is bounded by the lower coronary ligament and below by the general peritoneal cavity.

- The space extends from the lateral abdominal wall to the lesser sac and foramen of Winslow medially.

- The inferoposterior surface of the liver forms the anterior margin of the space, which is limited posteriorly by the right kidney and the hepatic flexure of the colon.

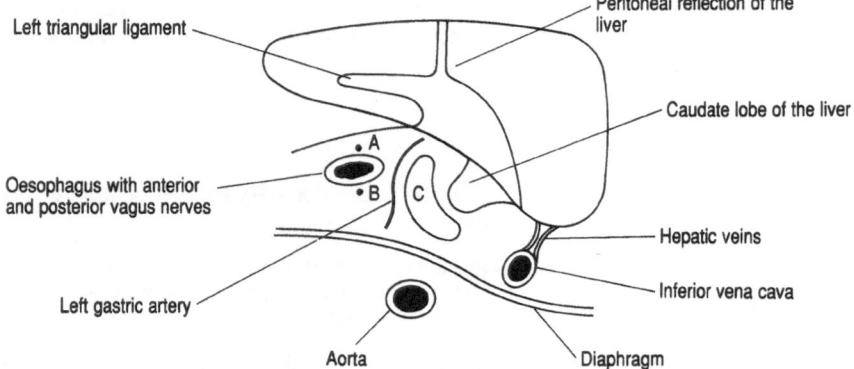

FIG. C *Transverse section through the upper abdomen. A and B, anterior and posterior vagus nerves; C, upper recess of the lesser sac.*

Left Posterior Subphrenic Space: Lesser Sac (fig. c)

- This space lies between the diaphragm, liver and stomach.

- The lateral boundary is the inferior vena cava with the abdominal portion of the oesophagus medially.

- Anteroposteriorly the space extends from the caudate lobe of the liver to the right crus of the diaphragm and the thoracic aorta.

Splenectomy

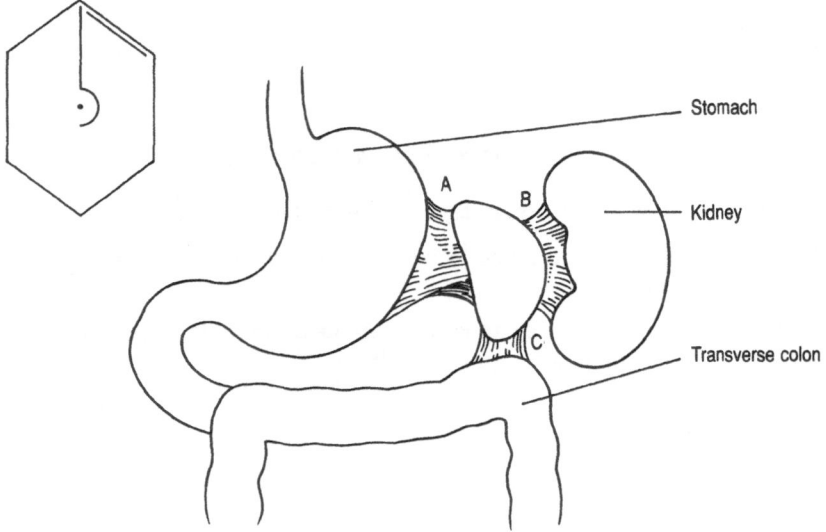

FIG. A *Spleen and ligamentous attachments. A, gastrosplenic; B, lienorenal; and C, adhesion to splenic flexure of colon.*

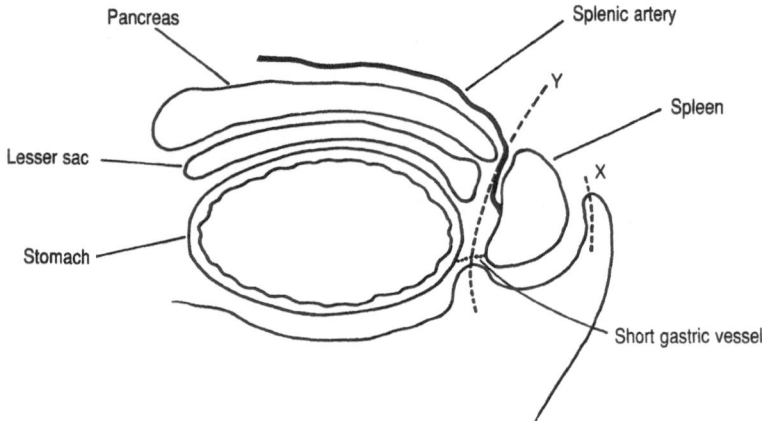

FIG. B *Transverse section through the stomach to show relations of the spleen to the pancreas, lesser sac, gastrosplenic and lienorenal ligaments. X, Division (- - -), lienorenal ligament. Y, Division, gastrosplenic ligament containing the short gastric vessels (. . .).*

The size of the spleen to be removed affects the approach to the operation. As the spleen enlarges it may become adherent to the underside of the diaphragm, the stomach and splenic flexure of the colon. For very large spleens a thoraco-abdominal approach may therefore be required. The splenic artery and vein run in continuity from the hilum along the upper border of the pancreas. There is only a space of some 2 cm between the hilum and the tail of the pancreas and care is required to avoid pancreatic injury. Accessory spleens (splenunculi) may be present and should be preserved if the spleen is being removed for trauma. However, in conditions such as lymphoma and myelofibrosis, where hypersplenism and extramedullary haemopoiesis may occur, it is important to remove accessory splenic tissue.

- Division of the lienorenal ligament allows medial and anterior displacement of the spleen so that it can be retracted into the wound (fig. a).

- The attachment of the upper, medial surface of the spleen to the stomach is severed by dividing the short gastric vessels in the gastrosplenic ligament (fig. a). In performing this manoeuvre care must be taken to avoid accidental clamping of the stomach wall.

- It should now be possible to identify clearly the tail of the pancreas and the splenic artery and splenic vein (fig. b). They can then be individually divided and ligated allowing the spleen to be removed.

- The diaphragm and splenic flexure of the colon should be carefully inspected for tears after removal of a large, adherent spleen.

Partial Pancreatectomy (Whipple's Operation)

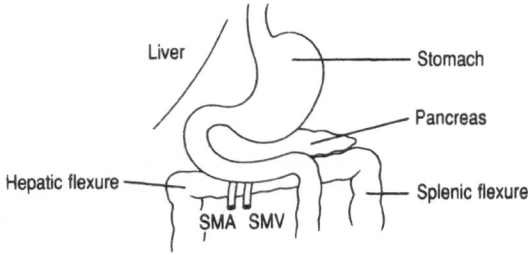

FIG. A *Posterior relations of the duodenum. SMA, superior mesenteric artery; SMV, superior mesenteric vein.*

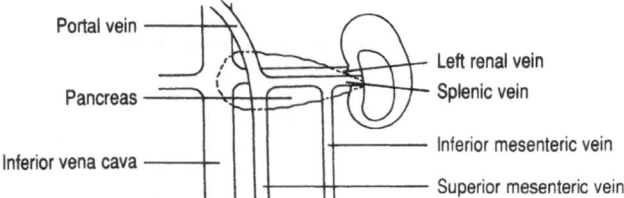

FIG. B *Posterior relations of the pancreas.*

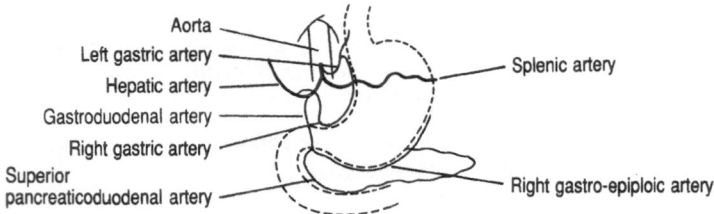

FIG. C *Arterial blood supply to the gastric antrum and the head of pancreas.*

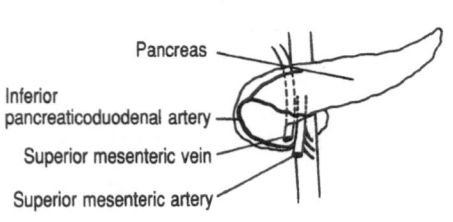

FIG. D *Blood supply of the pancreatic head.*

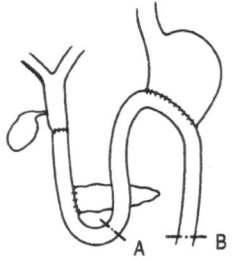

FIG. E *Reconstruction after partial pancreatectomy. Alternatively A can be sewn to B to create a Roux-en-Y.*

Partial Pancreatectomy (Whipple's Operation)

This procedure is carried out for carcinoma of the ampulla of Vater and cholangiocarcinomas at the lower end of the common bile duct. Carcinomas of the head of the pancreas are usually too extensive for a Whipple's operation to be curative. The procedure is impossible if tumour growth has spread to involve the portal vein at the junction between the head and body of the gland.

- The duodenum is exposed by mobilising the hepatic flexure (fig. a) and dividing its peritoneal reflections.

- The common bile duct, lying in the free edge of the lesser omentum, is identified above the duodenum and mobilised for later transection. Care should be taken to avoid damage to the inferiorly situated portal vein (fig. b).

- The superior mesenteric vein passes behind the pancreas to join the splenic vein to form the portal vein (fig. b). A plane of dissection is developed along the anterior surface of the superior mesenteric vein, separating it from the pancreas. Medially small venous tributaries, which join the superior mesenteric vein and portal vein from the head of the pancreas, require careful ligation.

- The right gastric, gastroduodenal and gastro-epiploic vessels are divided and ligated (fig. c). This allows the pyloric antrum to be mobilised and divided. The first and second parts of the duodenum can then be mobilised by incising the lateral peritoneal fold (Kocher's manoeuvre) and separating the duodenum from the underlying inferior vena cava.

- The inferior pancreaticoduodenal artery is divided as it branches from the superior mesenteric artery (fig. d). This artery divides into anterior and posterior branches as does the superior pancreaticoduodenal artery, which thus forms a double loop of vessels between the pancreatic head and the second part of the duodenum (fig. d).

- Following excision of the specimen reconstruction can be achieved by serial anastomoses between the jejunum and the stomach, the common bile duct and the distal end of the pancreas (fig. e).

Appendicectomy

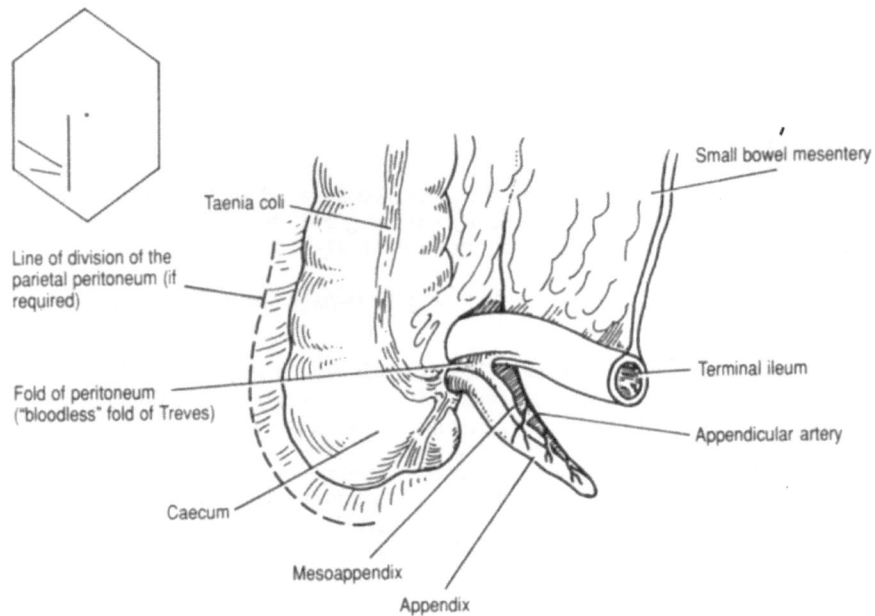

Taenia coli

Line of division of the
parietal peritoneum (if
required)

Fold of peritoneum
("bloodless" fold of Treves)

Caecum

Mesoappendix

Appendix

Small bowel mesentery

Terminal ileum

Appendicular artery

FIG. A   *Relations and blood supply of the vermiform*
appendix.

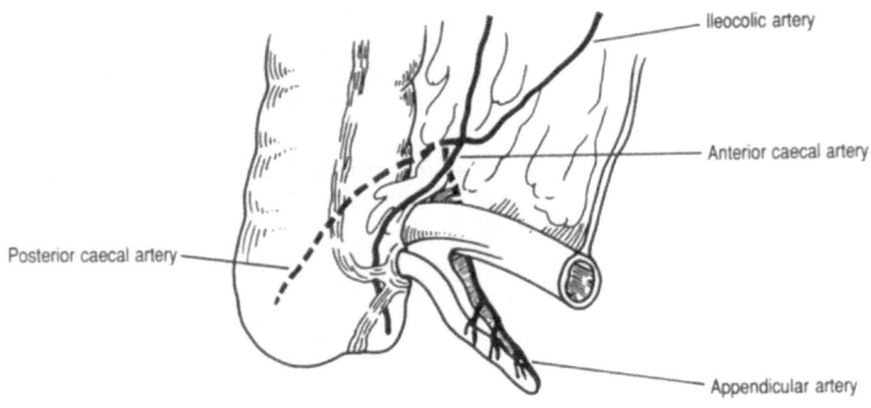

Posterior caecal artery

Ileocolic artery

Anterior caecal artery

Appendicular artery

FIG. B   *Relations and details of blood supply of the*
vermiform appendix.

The vermiform appendix arises from the caecum approximately 3 cm below the ileocaecal valve. The appendix may lie in a variety of positions. Paracolic and retrocaecal positions are the most common.

- The mesoappendix (fig. a) contains the appendicular artery, a branch of the posterior caecal artery, which in turn arises from the ileocolic artery (fig. b).

- The taenia coli converge at the base of the appendix. This often aids identification when the appendix has perforated and an abscess has formed (fig. a).

- When the appendix lies in the retrocaecal position it may be difficult to mobilise through the traditional gridiron incision. In this situation it may be necessary to extend the wound upwards to allow mobilisation of the caecum by division of the right lateral border of the parietal peritoneum (fig. a).

- It is advisable to bury the stump of the appendix to avoid the uncommon but troublesome problem of a faecal fistula.

Right Hemicolectomy

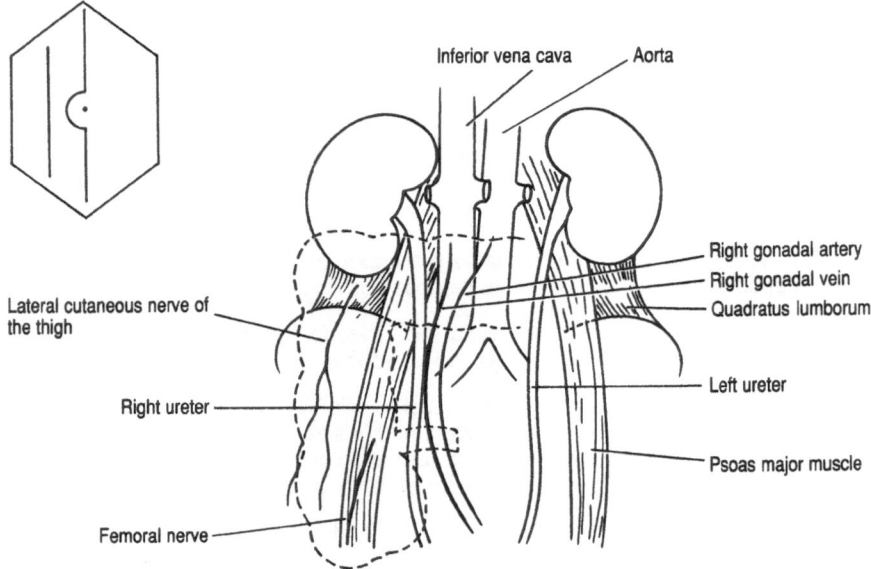

FIG. A *Posterior relations of the right side of the colon and caecum (– – –)*

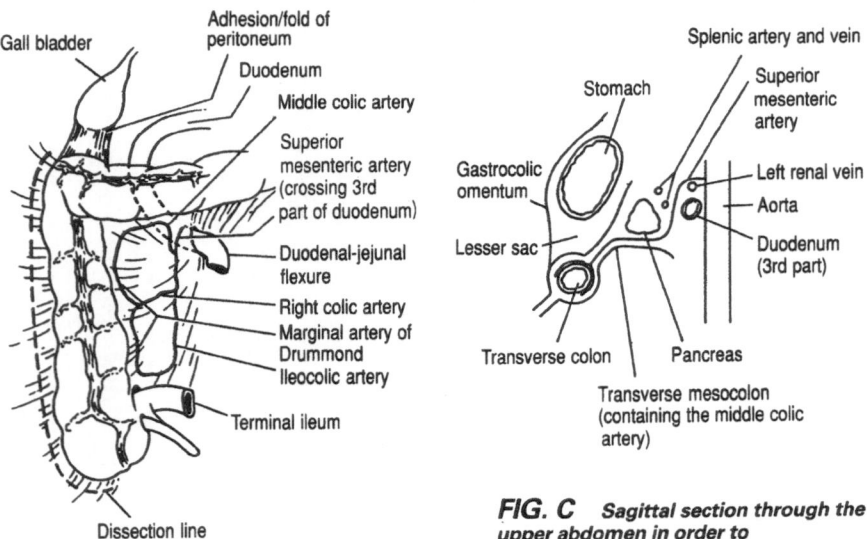

FIG. B *Upper relations of the right side of the colon and blood supply.*

FIG. C *Sagittal section through the upper abdomen in order to demonstrate the course of the superior mesenteric artery and its branches (middle colic artery).*

Right hemicolectomy for large bowel carcinoma requires removal of the mesentery and lymph node drainage in the territory of the ileocolic artery. This necessitates removal of at least 10 cm of terminal ileum, the caecum, the ascending colon and the proximal third of the transverse colon. In operations for non-malignant conditions, for example Crohn's disease and angiodysplasia of the ascending colon, more limited resections may be possible when the main trunk of the ileocolic artery is preserved. The psoas and iliacus muscles lie behind the caecum along with the lateral cutaneous nerve of the thigh and the femoral nerve. The right ureter and the accompanying gonadal vessels lie posteromedial to the ascending colon (fig. a) and must be positively identified during the operation. The hepatic flexure is related superiorly to the liver and posteriorly to the gall bladder and the lower pole of the right kidney. The proximal portion of the transverse colon is closely applied to the junction of the second and third parts of the duodenum (fig. b).

- The parietal peritoneal fold, situated along the lateral border of the caecum and ascending colon, is divided so that a retroperitoneal plane can be developed behind the large bowel. At this point the ureter and gonadal vessels are identified and kept in view throughout the dissection (figs. a and b).

- As the dissection proceeds upwards the hepatic flexure and transverse colon are carefully separated from the underlying duodenum (figs. b and c).

- Following the resection the blood supply to the colonic end of the anastomosis will be maintained by a supply from the marginal artery of Drummond. This vessel runs along the medial border of the colon and is supplied by branches from the middle colic, right colic and ileocolic arteries (fig. b).

Left Hemicolectomy

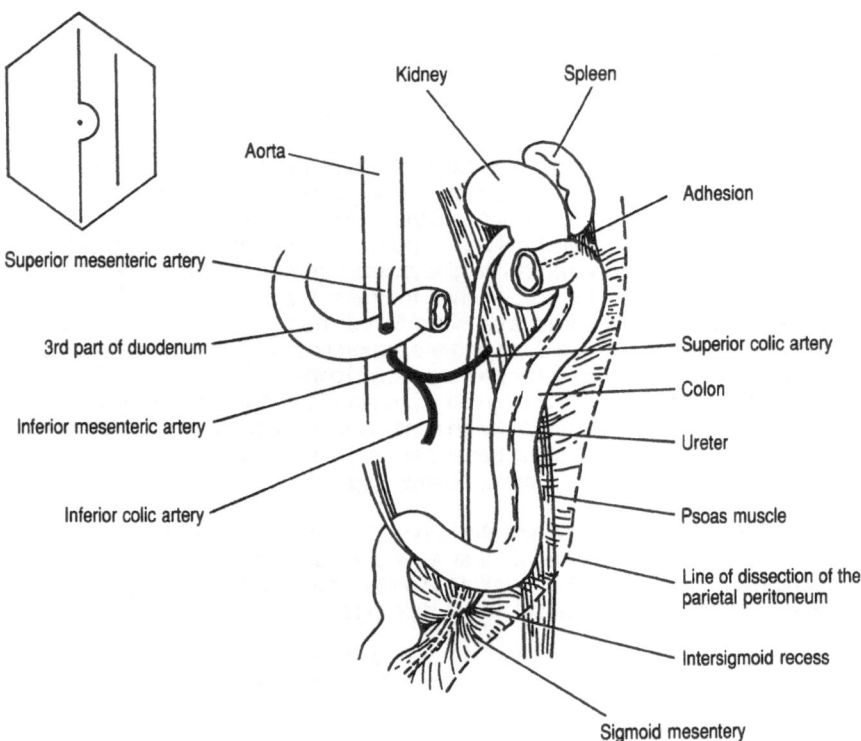

Kidney

Spleen

Aorta

Adhesion

Superior mesenteric artery

3rd part of duodenum

Superior colic artery

Colon

Inferior mesenteric artery

Ureter

Inferior colic artery

Psoas muscle

Line of dissection of the parietal peritoneum

Intersigmoid recess

Sigmoid mesentery

FIG. A *The left side of the colon and its relations.*

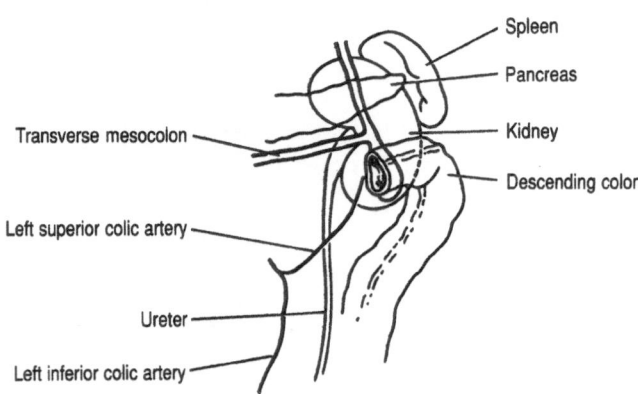

Spleen

Pancreas

Transverse mesocolon

Kidney

Descending colon

Left superior colic artery

Ureter

Left inferior colic artery

FIG. B *Structures posterior to the splenic flexure.*

Removal of the left side of the colon usually involves excision of the splenic flexure, descending colon and sigmoid colon. If the operation is undertaken for carcinoma an en bloc removal of the mesentery and lymph nodes with flush ligation of the inferior mesenteric artery at its origin from the aorta will be required. The blood supply to the subsequent colonic anastomosis is maintained by the marginal artery of Drummond. This vessel is supplied superiorly by the middle colic artery (a branch of the superior mesenteric artery) and inferiorly by the superior haemorrhoidal vessels (terminal branches of the internal iliac artery). The splenic flexure of the colon is often adherent to the splenic capsule and care must be taken to avoid capsular tears (fig. a). The left ureter can be found in the intersigmoid recess at the apex of the sigmoid mesentery (fig. a). The left ureter lies just lateral to the abdominal aorta, running laterally to cross the common iliac artery at its bifurcation.

- Mobilisation of the splenic flexure by division of the parietal peritoneum lateral to the colon enables division of any adhesions to the spleen (fig. a).

- The inferior mesenteric artery branches off from the aorta at the level of L3. The vessel should be identified, divided and ligated at an early stage in the operative procedure. It divides into the left superior and inferior colic branches (fig. b). These branches anastomose with the splenic branch of the middle colic artery and the superior haemorrhoidal vessels; the latter are derived from the internal iliac arteries respectively.

- As the sigmoid colon and descending colon are drawn forward the left ureter and gonadal vessels should be positively identified and then maintained in view throughout the procedure (figs. a and b).

- Because of the tenuous vascularity of the colon an end-to-end anastomosis must not be performed under tension. Therefore adequate colonic mobilisation and preservation of the marginal blood supply are vitally important principles.

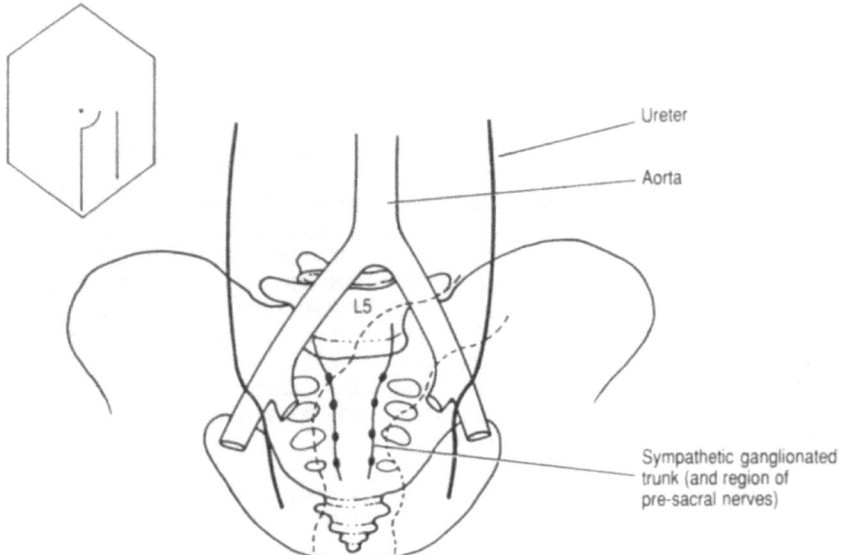

FIG. A *Posterior relations of the rectum (– – –) denotes rectum.*

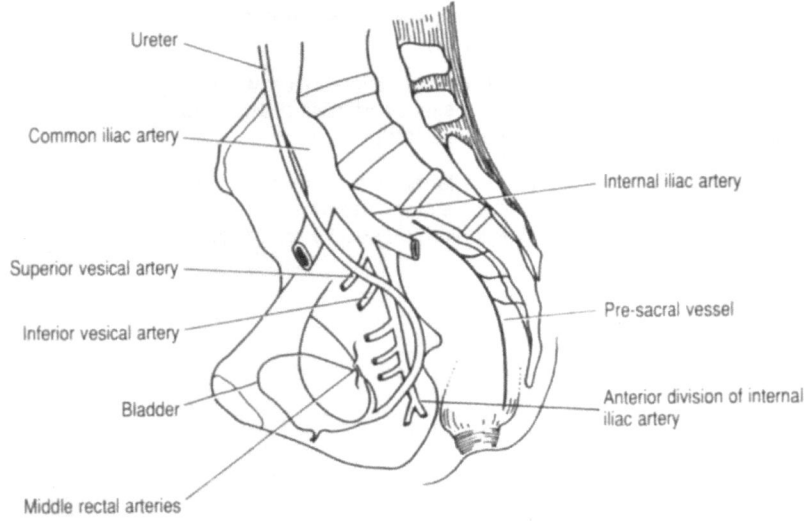

FIG. B *Lateral relations of the rectum.*

The rectum is part of the hind gut, extending from the pelvic colon to the anal canal. An anterior longitudinal band of muscle extends along the length of the rectum forming the rectourethralis muscle, passing to the external urethral sphincter and the perineal body. The upper part of the rectum receives its arterial blood supply from the left inferior colic artery and the superior rectal artery, both distal branches of the inferior mesenteric artery. The body of the rectum and the anal canal are supplied by the middle and inferior rectal vessels, which are terminal branches of the internal iliac arteries (figs. a and b). The anorectal junction formed by the puborectalis muscle is at the level of the levator ani muscles which surround and support the rectum forming the pelvic floor.

Venous drainage of the lower rectum and anal canal is via the inferior and middle rectal veins to the systemic circulation via the internal iliac veins. The upper part of the rectum is drained by the superior rectal vein, which is a tributary of the inferior mesenteric vein. The rectal plexus of veins allows a free communication between the portal and systemic venous systems. Above the anorectal junction the drainage runs in the mesentery to connect with the pre-aortic nodes around the origin of the inferior mesenteric artery. Lymphatics in the perianal region drain to the inguinal region, which explains why anal tumours may present with secondary spread to the groin nodes. Peritoneum only covers the upper and middle thirds of the rectum, turning forwards anteriorly to form the rectovesical pouch in the male and the pouch of Douglas in the female (fig. b). On each side of the rectum the peritoneum is reflected over the lateral walls of the pelvis, covering the iliac vessels and the ureter.

- Identifying both ureters and their passage into the pelvis is an important first step in the operative procedure. The left ureter is identified first when the sigmoid colon has been mobilised by dividing the white line where the sigmoid mesentery is attached to the parietal peritoneum and the lateral abdominal wall. The right ureter is identified as the peritoneum at the rectosigmoid junction on the right side of the colon is incised.

- These initial incisions allow the pre-sacral space to be opened and the posterior aspect of the rectum mobilised. Care must be taken at this stage to avoid damage to the pre-sacral nerves (fig. a).

- Vigorous blunt dissection of the rectum may cause trauma to the pre-sacral nerves and bleeding from the pre-sacral veins. This bleeding may be difficult to control due to retraction of the vessels into the sacrum (fig. b).

- For most anterior resection procedures it is sufficient to divide the fold of peritoneum running across the rectovesical pouch. If more extensive dissection of the rectum is required the steps described in the section on abdominoperineal excision of the rectum should be followed (p. 46).

Abdominoperineal Excision of the Rectum

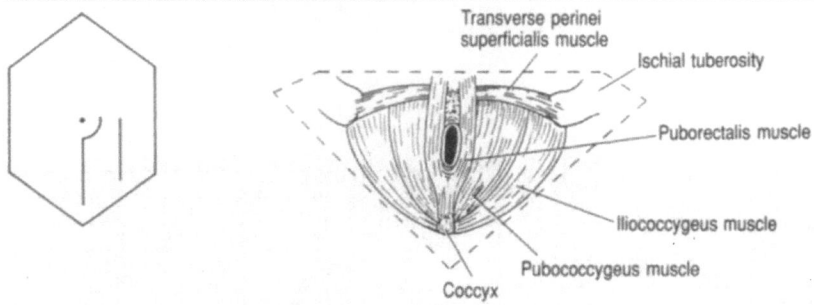

Transverse perinei
superficialis muscle

Ischial tuberosity

Puborectalis muscle

Iliococcygeus muscle

Pubococcygeus muscle

Coccyx

FIG. A *Inferior aspect of the pelvic
floor (anal triangle ▽).*

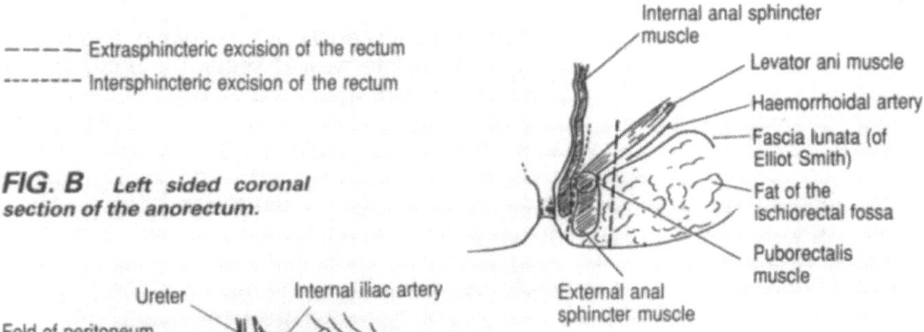

---- Extrasphincteric excision of the rectum

------- Intersphincteric excision of the rectum

FIG. B *Left sided coronal
section of the anorectum.*

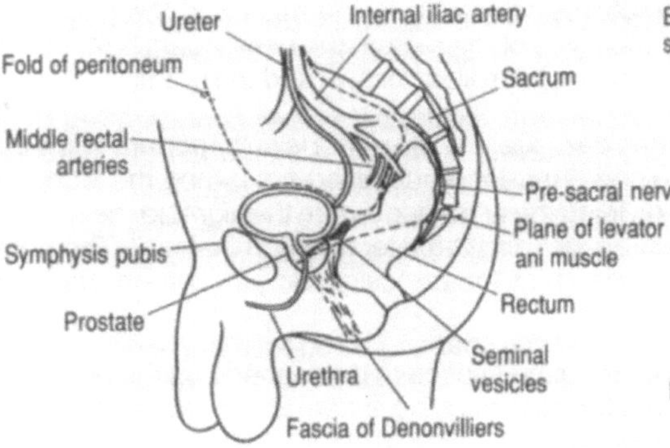

Internal anal sphincter
muscle

Levator ani muscle

Haemorrhoidal artery

Fascia lunata (of
Elliot Smith)

Fat of the
ischiorectal fossa

Puborectalis
muscle

External anal
sphincter muscle

Ureter

Internal iliac artery

Fold of peritoneum

Middle rectal
arteries

Sacrum

Symphysis pubis

Prostate

Pre-sacral nerve

Plane of levator
ani muscle

Rectum

Urethra

Seminal
vesicles

Fascia of Denonvilliers

FIG. C *Anterolateral relations of
the rectum in the male.*

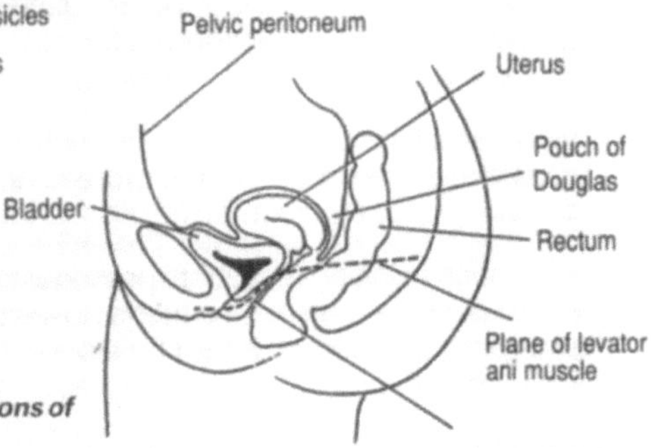

Pelvic peritoneum

Uterus

Pouch of
Douglas

Bladder

Rectum

Plane of levator
ani muscle

FIG. D *Anterolateral relations of
the rectum in the female.*

Abdominoperineal Excision of the Rectum

Mobilisation of the rectum is performed as for anterior resection (see p. 44). The perineum is a diamond-shaped space between the symphysis pubis anteriorly and the coccyx posteriorly, bounded anterolaterally by the ischiopubic rami, laterally by the ischial tuberosities and posterolaterally by the lower borders of the sacrotuberous ligaments (fig. a). It is artificially divided by a line joining the ischial tuberosities into the anal and urogenital triangles (fig. a). The anorectum can be excised between the internal and external anal sphincters (intersphincteric) or outside the external anal sphincter (extrasphincteric) (fig. b). The choice of procedure depends upon the pathology, intersphincteric dissection being used for inflammatory bowel disease and extrasphincteric for carcinoma.

Extrasphincteric Excision of the Rectum

- Posteriorly the pubococcygeus muscle is divided (fig. a) to allow access to the pre-sacral space, facilitating synchronous excision in liaison with the abdominal operator.

- Anteriorly the plane of dissection should remain behind the transverse perinei superficialis and transverse perinei profundus muscles (fig. a). In the male this will ensure that the urethra is not damaged. The fascia of Denonvilliers is the correct plane to advance along anteriorly in the male (fig. c).

- Laterally each ischiorectal fossa is opened allowing visualisation of the levator ani muscles. This is achieved by dividing the pubococcygeus and ischiococcygeus muscles (figs. a and b).

- The vagina lies adjacent to the rectum in the female and its posterior wall may have to be excised with the rectum if there is tumour invasion (fig. d).

Intersphincteric Excision of the Rectum

- This rectal excision technique leaves the external anal sphincter in place by the development of a plane between the internal and external anal sphincters (fig. b).

Stomas

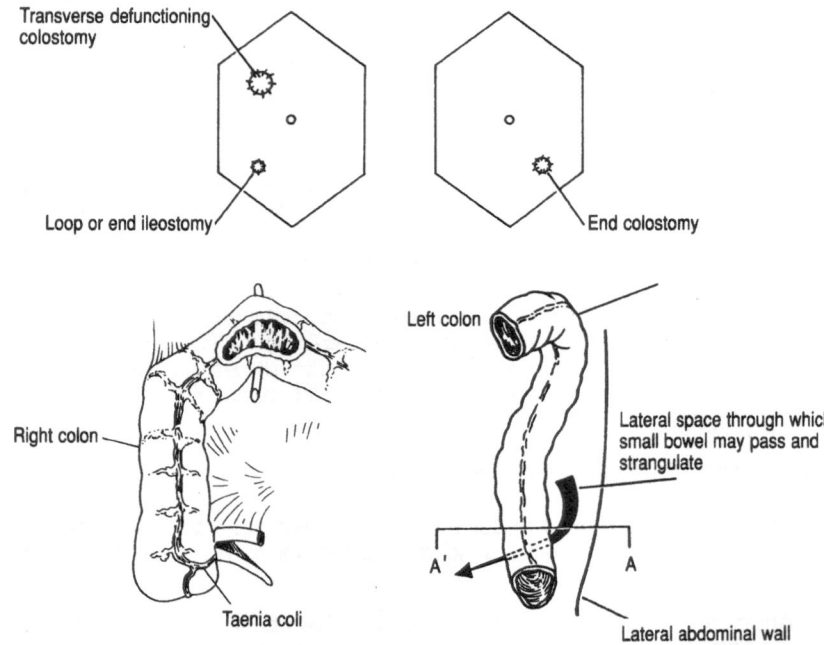

Transverse defunctioning colostomy

Loop or end ileostomy

End colostomy

Left colon

Lateral space through which small bowel may pass and strangulate

Right colon

A'

A

Taenia coli

Lateral abdominal wall

FIG. A *Transverse colostomy, ileostomy and sites.*

FIG. B *Descending colon and colostomy site.*

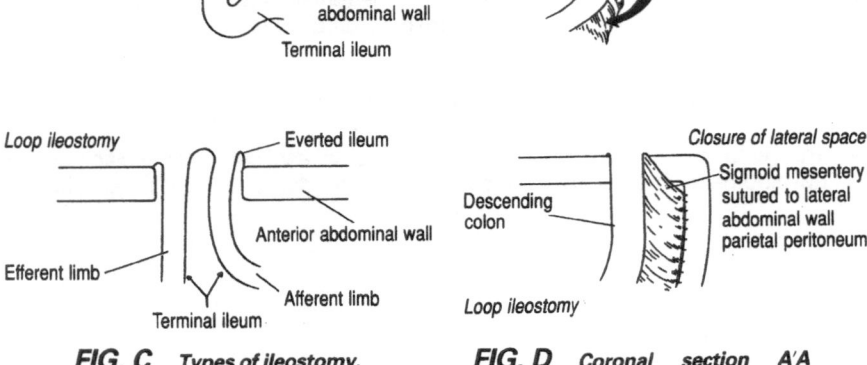

Brooke's end ileostomy

Everted ileum

Anterior abdominal wall

Terminal ileum

Descending colon

Loop ileostomy

Everted ileum

Anterior abdominal wall

Efferent limb

Afferent limb

Terminal ileum

Descending colon

Loop ileostomy

Closure of lateral space

Sigmoid mesentery sutured to lateral abdominal wall parietal peritoneum

FIG. C *Types of ileostomy.*

FIG. D *Coronal section A'A through the abdomen to demonstrate closing the lateral space.*

Many anatomical factors contribute to the successful formation of a stoma: placement on the anterior abdominal wall, avoidance of damage to the mesentery, and adequate trephine through the anterior abdominal wall.

- Figure a demonstrates the site of a transverse defunctioning colostomy. The bowel is opened on the ante-mesenteric border, along the taenia coli for approximately 5 cm. Care should be taken not to damage the transverse mesocolon when making a small hole beneath the bowel for the placement of the rod for temporary loop support.

- During the formation of an end colostomy (fig. b) it is important to close the lateral space to prevent small bowel strangulation (fig. c).

- An end ileostomy should be fashioned so that a spout is formed to prevent excoriation of the surrounding skin (fig. d). When a loop ileostomy is fashioned the afferent limb can be everted whilst the efferent limb is not (fig. d). Also, it is more helpful to the patient if the afferent limb in a loop ileostomy is situated inferiorly (dependently) so that effluent collection is aided in the upright ambulatory position.

Haemorrhoidectomy

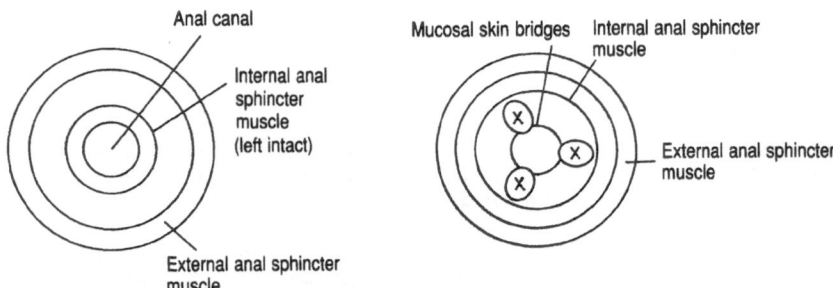

FIG. A   *Sites of haemorrhoids. X = sites of ligation of haemorrhoids.*

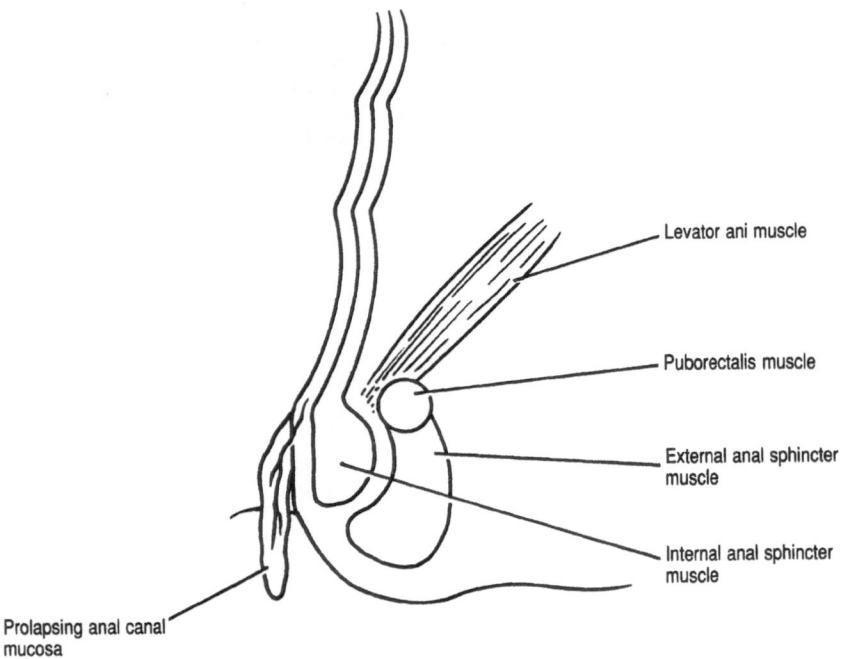

FIG. B   *Coronal section through left anorectal region.*

Haemorrhoidectomy is performed for the treatment of third-degree haemorrhoids. The haemorrhoids are usually situated at 3, 7 and 11 o'clock (mirroring the pattern of venous drainage) when the patient is in the lithotomy position (fig. a).

- It is very important to leave bridges between skin and mucosa in continuity between the regions of mucosal excision, otherwise there will be healing by cicatrisation resulting in anal canal stenosis (fig. a).

- When the mucosa is incised the circular pale muscle of the internal anal sphincter should be identified so that it is not accidentally incised, excised or transfixed when ligating the base of the haemorrhoids (fig. b).

Perianal Sepsis, Abscess and Fistulae

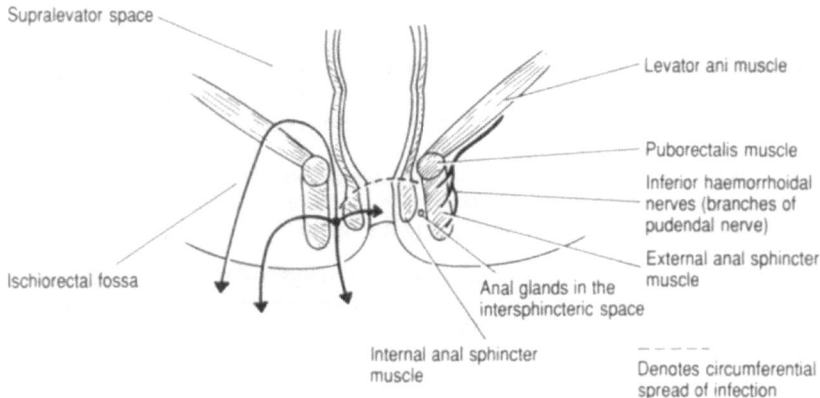

Supralevator space

Levator ani muscle

Puborectalis muscle

Inferior haemorrhoidal nerves (branches of pudendal nerve)

External anal sphincter muscle

Ischiorectal fossa

Anal glands in the intersphincteric space

Internal anal sphincter muscle

Denotes circumferential spread of infection

FIG. A   *Coronal section of the anorectal region showing ways of spread of infection and the development of fistulae.*

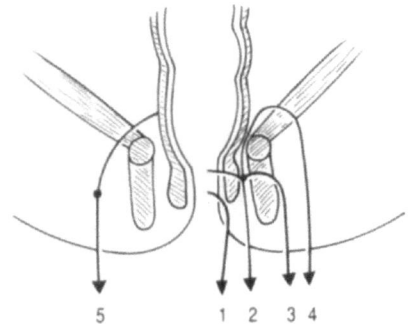

5   1 2   3 4

FIG. B   *Coronal section of the anorectal region as for FIG. A, demonstrating the different types of perianal fistulae: 1, superficial (no sphincter muscle involved); 2, intersphincteric; 3, transsphincteric; 4, supralevator; 5, extrasphincteric.*

Perianal Sepsis, Abscess and Fistulae

The treatment of perianal sepsis and fistulae depends primarily upon the accurate anatomical delineation of the fistulous tracks and related abscess cavities (figs. a and b). Usually infection/abscess formation occurs in the anal glands which lie in the intersphincteric space (fig. a).

- Figure b demonstrates the various sites of infection and fistulous tracts which can occur. In the majority of cases the fistulous tract can be laid open (fistulotomy). However, if fistulotomy were performed for supralevator fistulae, serious damage to the anorectal sphincter musculature would result.

- The inferior haemorrhoidal nerves, branches of the pudendal nerve, enter the external anal sphincter laterally and may consequently be inadvertently damaged by fistula and/or abscess surgery (fig. a).

- If a straightforward abscess is present then it should be deroofed, again being careful not to include in the incision any part of the sphincter apparatus.

Inguinal Herniae

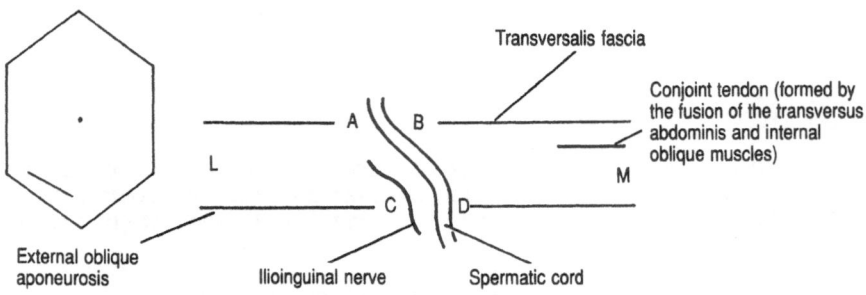

FIG. A *The inguinal canal from above in transverse section (AB deep and CD superficial inguinal ring).*

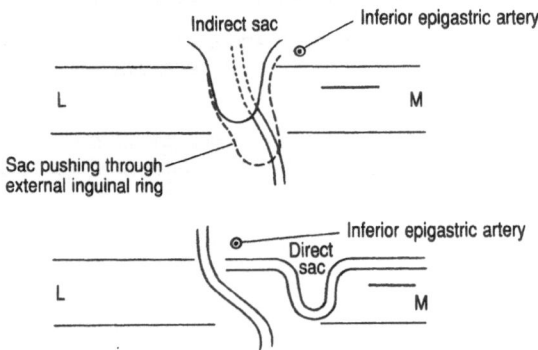

FIG. B *Different positions of indirect and direct herniae sacs. L, lateral; M, medial.*

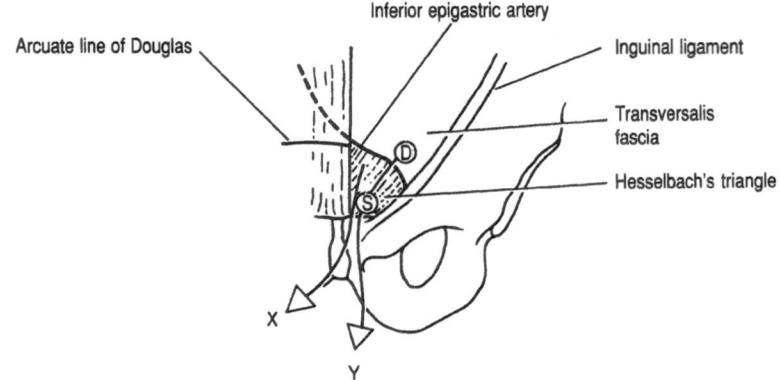

FIG. C *Left groin showing the deep (D) and superficial (S) inguinal rings; X and Y direct and indirect, inguinal herniae sacs.*

The inguinal canal is an oblique passage through the anterior abdominal wall. It extends from the deep inguinal ring, a defect in the transversalis fascia, to the superficial inguinal ring, an oval opening in the external oblique aponeurosis (figs a. and b). The inguinal canal in the adult is 4 cm long and is directed downwards, forwards and medially (fig. a). In the child (under 5 years of age) the deep and superficial rings are in direct alignment.

The anterior wall of the inguinal canal is formed by the aponeurosis of the external oblique muscle while the posterior wall is formed by the transversalis fascia in the entire length of the canal and the conjoint tendon in the medial half (fig. a). The roof is formed by the arched lower border of the internal oblique and transversus abdominis muscles. The floor is formed predominantly by the free edge of the inguinal ligament.

The spermatic cord extends from the deep inguinal ring to the posterosuperior border of the testicle. It is bounded by the external spermatic fascia, cremaster muscle and the internal spermatic fascia, which are derived from the external oblique aponeurosis, internal oblique muscle and the transversalis fascia respectively. These layers surround the vas deferens and its vessels. The testicular artery rises from the abdominal aorta, lies anteriorly on the vas and is often covered by spermatic veins.

The genital branch of the genitofemoral nerve (L1 and L2) (fig. a) supplies the cremaster muscle and gives a sensory branch to the tunica vaginalis.

The inguinal canal transmits the ilioinguinal nerve (anterior primary ramus of L2) (fig. a). This nerve passes between the transversus abdominis and internal oblique muscles, eventually piercing the internal oblique muscle to pass into the inguinal canal (fig. a).

- In an indirect inguinal hernia the deep ring is lax and a hernial sac pushes into the inguinal canal (fig. b). A direct inguinal hernial sac lies medial to the inferior epigastric artery and pushes its way through the transversalis fascia in Hesselbach's triangle (figs. b and c).

- An indirect sac is nearly always situated on top of the spermatic cord in the male or the round ligament of the uterus in the female (fig. b).

- An indirect sac is treated by herniotomy and herniorrhaphy. There are a number of different repairs but the principle is to plicate the internal deep ring and transversalis fascia while strengthening the posterior wall of the inguinal canal with a non-absorbable suture.

- A direct sac is treated as above except without a herniotomy.

Femoral Hernia

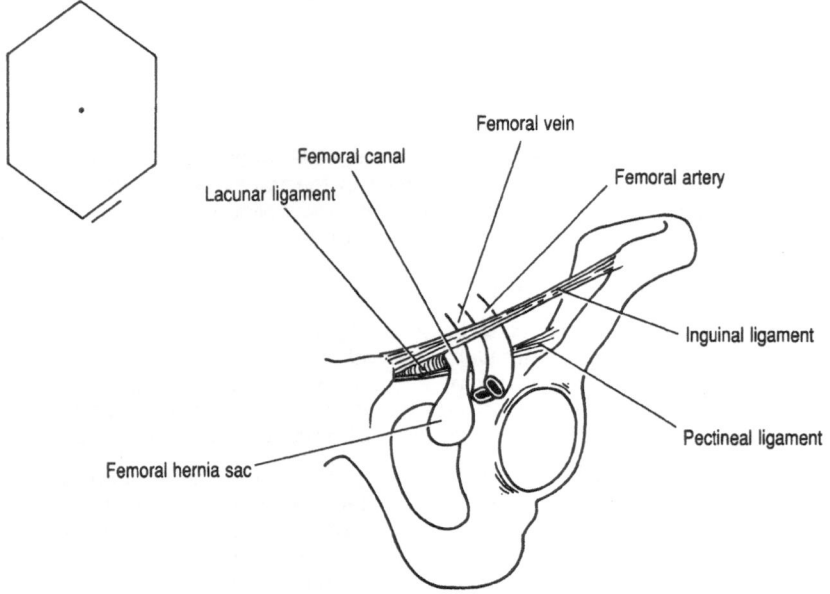

FIG. A   *Femoral hernia sac and related ligaments.*

Femoral vein

Femoral canal

Femoral artery

Lacunar ligament

Inguinal ligament

Pectineal ligament

Femoral hernia sac

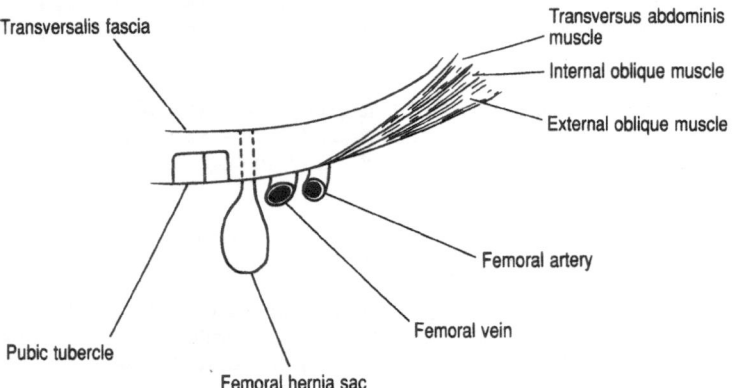

FIG. B   *Transverse section through left groin showing position of the femoral hernia sac and its relation to the femoral vessels.*

Transversalis fascia

Transversus abdominis muscle

Internal oblique muscle

External oblique muscle

Femoral artery

Femoral vein

Pubic tubercle

Femoral hernia sac

The femoral canal is medial to the femoral vein and lateral to the lacunar ligament (fig. a). It lies below the inguinal ligament; the pectineal ligament forms its posterior surface (fig. a). A femoral hernia therefore presents below and lateral to the pubic tubercle.

- The contents of the sac may include omentum, small bowel, ovary, fallopian tube and occasionally the appendix.

- When approaching the hernia from below care should be taken to avoid damage to the femoral vein when plication sutures are placed between the inguinal and pectineal ligaments (fig. a).

- In the McEvedy operation an oblique incision is made above the inguinal ligament, the rectus sheath is incised along its lateral border and the neck of the sac defined after dividing the transversalis fascia (fig. b). With the sac reduced the defect can be clearly visualised from above and repaired with interrupted sutures.

III. Vasculature

Abdominal Aortic Aneurysm (Infra-renal)

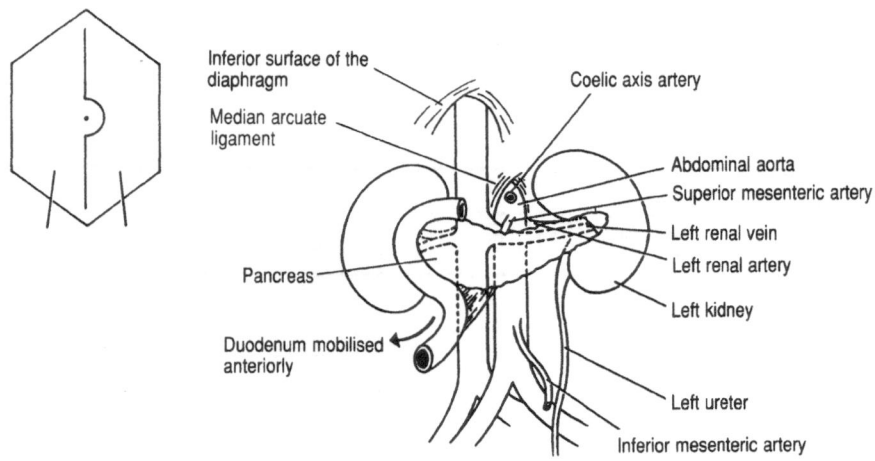

Inferior surface of the diaphragm

Coelic axis artery

Median arcuate ligament

Abdominal aorta

Superior mesenteric artery

Left renal vein

Pancreas

Left renal artery

Left kidney

Duodenum mobilised anteriorly

Left ureter

Inferior mesenteric artery

FIG. A *Anterior relations of the abdominal aorta.*

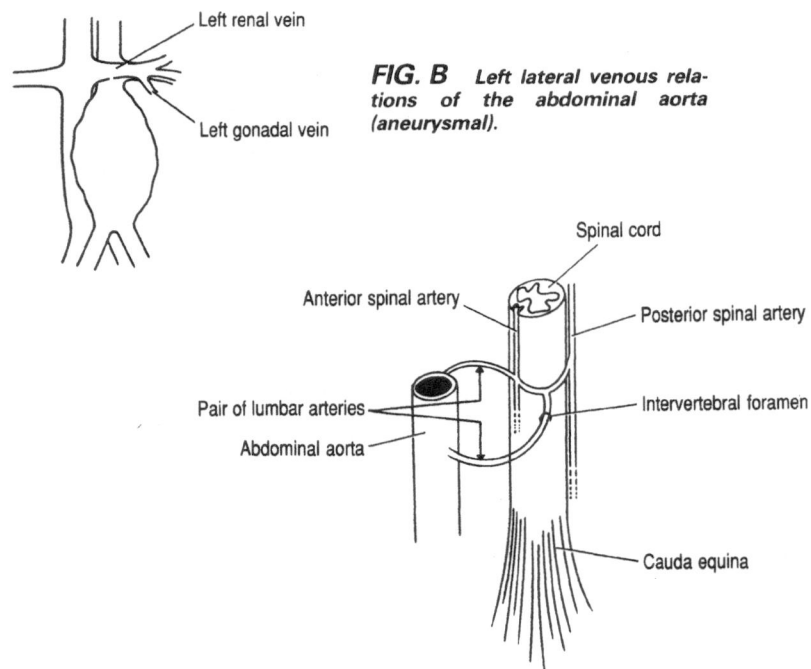

Left renal vein

FIG. B *Left lateral venous relations of the abdominal aorta (aneurysmal).*

Left gonadal vein

Spinal cord

Anterior spinal artery

Posterior spinal artery

Pair of lumbar arteries

Intervertebral foramen

Abdominal aorta

Cauda equina

FIG. C *Anastomotic connections between aortic lumbar arteries and the anterior and posterior spinal arteries.*

Abdominal Aortic Aneurysm (Infra-renal)

The abdominal aorta begins at the lower border of the 12th thoracic vertebra and extends from the median arcuate ligament to its site of bifurcation opposite the 4th lumbar vertebra (fig. a). Along its course it lies on the vertebral bodies, intervertebral discs and anterior longitudinal ligament.

- The first step in gaining access to the aorta is to divide the posterior peritoneum. Superiorly the incision passes between the duodenum medially and the inferior mesenteric vein laterally (fig. a). The duodeno–jejunal flexure can then be retracted upwards to achieve visualisation of the infra-renal portion of the aorta. The left renal vein is identified running across the aorta (figs. a and b). In mobilising the neck of the aneurysm sac care must be taken not to tear the gonadal vein which joins the inferior aspect of the left renal vein as shown in fig. b. In large aneurysms elective division of the left renal vein may be necessary to gain access to the neck of the aneurysm sac.

- Four pairs of lumbar arteries and veins arise from the posterior aspect of the aorta and the inferior vena cava (fig. c). The lumbar veins are thin-walled and particularly susceptible to damage during surgery for a ruptured or leaking aortic aneurysm where the operative field is obscured by haematoma.

- The lumbar arteries supply the spinal cord and cauda equina by travelling through the intervertebral foramina (fig. c). Paraplegia is a rare complication of repair and is thought to be due to interruption of the blood supply to the anterior spinal artery (the artery of Adamkiewicz) (fig. c).

- The left ureter lies close to the left lateral border of the aneurysm sac and may be adherent to it. Therefore the ureter should always be positively identified before excising any part of the aneurysm sac.

- Whether a tube graft or a bifurcation graft is applied, control of the common iliac arteries will be required. These vessels are closely applied to the underlying common iliac veins. Atherosclerotic or aneurysmal arteries may be quite densely adherent to these veins. Great care is therefore required during arterial mobilisation to avoid venous damage and the resulting major haemorrhage. In advanced aorto-iliac disease the inferior mesenteric artery is frequently occluded. However, if back flow is demonstrated the artery may be reimplanted into the aortic graft to preserve left colonic blood flow.

- In reconstructing the posterior abdominal wall structures the upper anastomotic line of the aortic repair should be covered by both aneurysm sac and parietal peritoneum. This prevents direct contact between the duodenum and the graft and consequently minimises the risk of aorto-enteric fistula.

- Retroperitoneal tunnelling to the groin is described in the next procedure (see Aortobifemoral Bypass Graft, p. 62).

Aortobifemoral Bypass Graft
(for occlusive arterial disease)

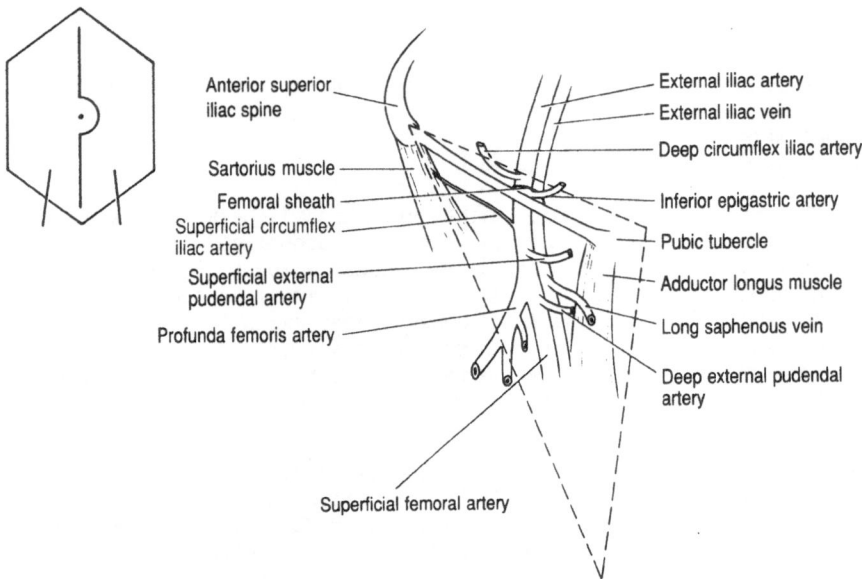

Anterior superior iliac spine

Sartorius muscle

Femoral sheath

Superficial circumflex iliac artery

Superficial external pudendal artery

Profunda femoris artery

External iliac artery

External iliac vein

Deep circumflex iliac artery

Inferior epigastric artery

Pubic tubercle

Adductor longus muscle

Long saphenous vein

Deep external pudendal artery

Superficial femoral artery

FIG. A *Contents of the right femoral triangle (– – –) lying underneath the fascia lata of the thigh.*

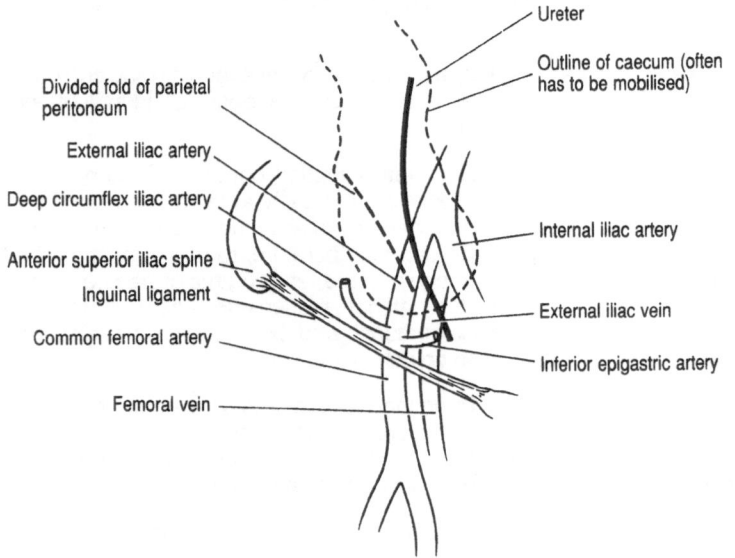

Ureter

Outline of caecum (often has to be mobilised)

Divided fold of parietal peritoneum

External iliac artery

Deep circumflex iliac artery

Anterior superior iliac spine

Inguinal ligament

Common femoral artery

Femoral vein

Internal iliac artery

External iliac vein

Inferior epigastric artery

FIG. B *Important pelvic structures to consider when tunnelling the graft into the groin.*

Aortobifemoral bypass grafting is a procedure for the treatment of aorto-iliac occlusive arterial disease. Dissection of the aorta can proceed as for an abdominal aortic aneurysm, thereby fashioning a proximal end-to-end (graft to aorta) anastomosis. However, some surgeons prefer an onlay graft technique to avoid interfering with lumbar or inferior mesenteric arterial blood flow (i.e. the aorta is left undivided). The femoral triangle (Scarpa's triangle) is an area bounded by the inguinal ligament superiorly, sartorius muscle laterally and the medial border of adductor longus muscle medially (fig. a). The floor of this triangle, containing the femoral vessels, is formed by adductor longus, pectineus and iliopsoas muscles from medial to lateral respectively; its roof is formed by the fascia lata (deep fascia) of the thigh.

- The graft is passed from the pelvis into the groin in the direction of and above the external iliac artery avoiding the caecum. Care should be taken to avoid damage to the external iliac vein and avulsion of the deep and superficial circumflex iliac arteries, which are branches of the external iliac and common femoral arteries respectively (fig. a).

- The inferior epigastric artery where it crosses the external iliac vein (fig. a) may also be injured during passage of one of the limbs of the graft into the groin.

- On the left side the graft is passed from the pelvis into the groin in the same way. Care should be taken as above, passing the graft under the sigmoid colon.

- In the pelvis both ureters are at risk when the parietal peritoneum is picked up in order to burrow along the superior aspects of the external iliac arteries (fig. b).

- End-to-side anastomoses are usually fashioned onto the common femoral artery, making sure they are not under undue tension.

Exposure of the Femoral Artery

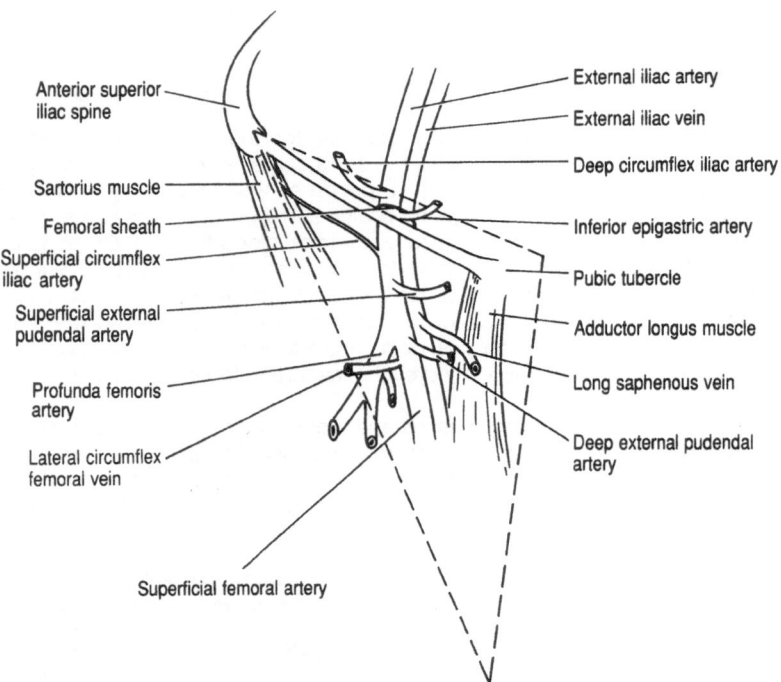

Anterior superior iliac spine

Sartorius muscle

Femoral sheath

Superficial circumflex iliac artery

Superficial external pudendal artery

Profunda femoris artery

Lateral circumflex femoral vein

External iliac artery

External iliac vein

Deep circumflex iliac artery

Inferior epigastric artery

Pubic tubercle

Adductor longus muscle

Long saphenous vein

Deep external pudendal artery

Superficial femoral artery

FIG. A *Contents of the right femoral triangle (– – –) underneath the fascia lata of the thigh.*

Exposure of the Femoral Artery

This dissection is common to all procedures involving the femoral artery: femoral embolectomy, distal anastomosis of an aortofemoral graft, femorofemoral bypass, profundoplasty and the upper anastomosis of a femoropopliteal graft.

- A vertical incision is made over the femoral artery extending as far as the inguinal ligament and if necessary curving laterally to provide adequate exposure.

- The femoral bifurcation is identified by observing the distinct change in calibre as the larger common femoral artery gives off the smaller superficial femoral artery.

- The profunda femoris artery arises from the posterolateral aspect of the common femoral artery (fig. a). In mobilising the profunda it is important to identify the lateral circumflex femoral vein which frequently runs across the profunda just distal to its origin. This vein runs directly into the femoral vein and if damaged can result in profuse haemorrhage.

Exposure of the Popliteal Artery

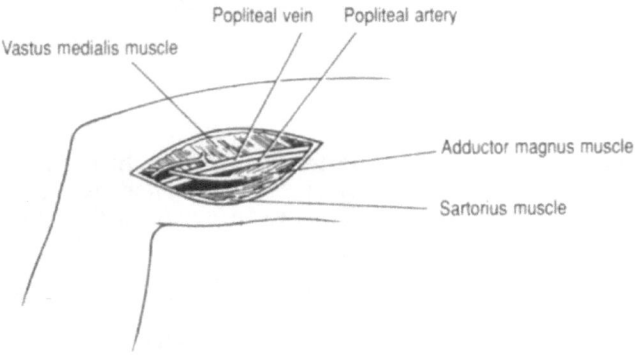

Vastus medialis muscle

Popliteal vein   Popliteal artery

Adductor magnus muscle

Sartorius muscle

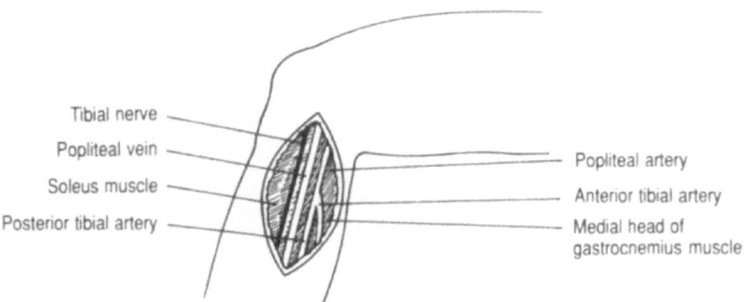

Tibial nerve

Popliteal vein

Soleus muscle

Posterior tibial artery

Popliteal artery

Anterior tibial artery

Medial head of gastrocnemius muscle

FIG. B *Medial below knee approach to the popliteal artery.*

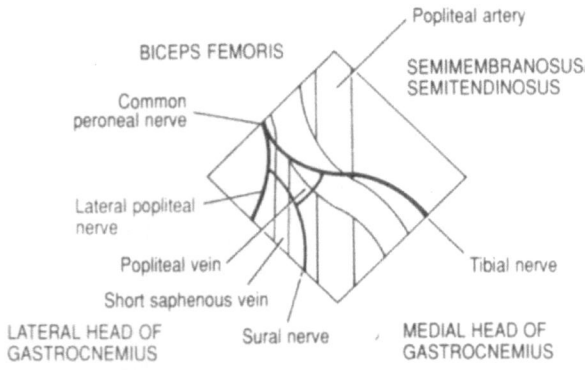

Popliteal artery

BICEPS FEMORIS

SEMIMEMBRANOSUS/ SEMITENDINOSUS

Common peroneal nerve

Lateral popliteal nerve

Popliteal vein

Short saphenous vein

Tibial nerve

LATERAL HEAD OF GASTROCNEMIUS

Sural nerve

MEDIAL HEAD OF GASTROCNEMIUS

FIG. C *Posterior aspect of the popliteal fossa and its boundaries.*

Exposure of the Popliteal Artery

Exposure of the popliteal artery is common to the following procedures: femoropopliteal bypass, distal embolectomy and ligation of a popliteal aneurysm. The popliteal artery descends from the opening in adductor magnus muscle to the lower border of the popliteus muscle. At this level it gives off the anterior tibial artery laterally. There is then a short tibioperoneal trunk before the artery finally divides into the peroneal and posterior tibial arteries.

Medial Approach

Above Knee

- The incision extends vertically from the medial femoral condyle upwards along the posterior border of vastus medialis muscle.

- Beneath the deep fascia of the thigh the sartorius muscle can be identified lying inferiorly and vastus medialis muscle superiorly (fig. a). On separation of these two muscles the popliteal artery can be exposed (superiorly the artery can be identified as it descends beneath the adductor magnus muscle).

- Above the knee the popliteal vein is lateral to the popliteal artery.

- Coursing under the surface of the sartorius muscle is the saphenous nerve, which can be damaged when retracting the sartorius muscle (fig. a).

Below Knee

- The incision extends from the medial tibial condyle down along the posterior border of the tibia.

- If the medial head of the gastrocnemius muscle is retracted inferiorly the popliteal vessels will be exposed (below the knee the popliteal vein is medial to the popliteal artery) (fig. b).

Posterior Approach

- A posterior sigmoid incision can be employed, the upper limb being medial in the thigh and the lower limb being lateral in the calf, with the two being connected by a horizontal incision turning across the flexure in the popliteal fossa (fig. c).

- The deep fascia overlying the popliteal fossa is divided in the midline, avoiding damage to the tibial and lateral popliteal nerves, sural nerve and short saphenous vein (fig. c).

Exposure of the Axillary Artery

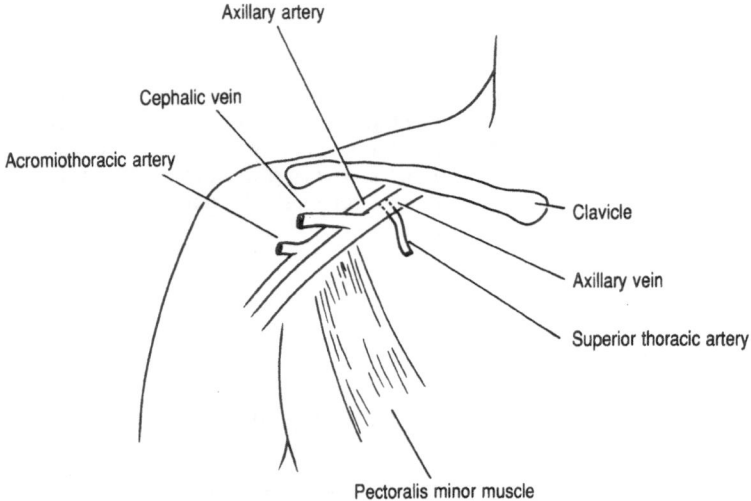

FIG. A *Relations of the first part of the axillary artery.*

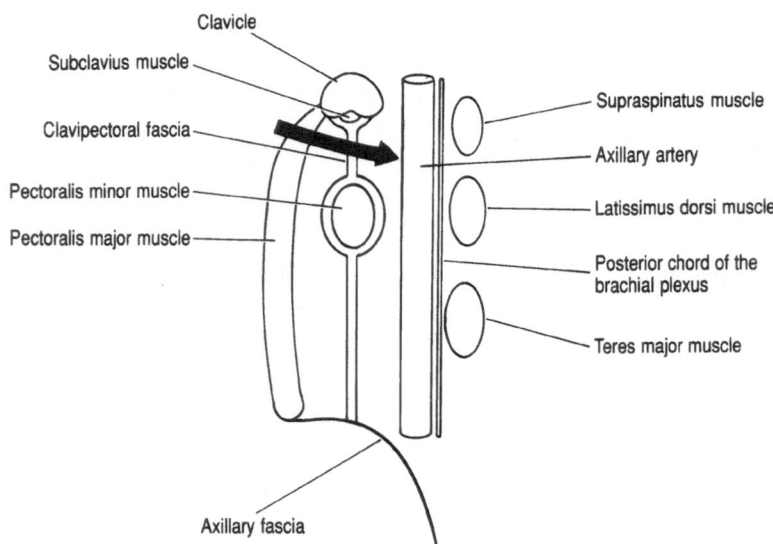

FIG. B *Sagittal section through the axilla showing the relations of the axillary artery and the approach to the first part (→).*

Exposure of the Axillary Artery

The axillary artery (Figs. a and b) is exposed for embolectomy and axillofemoral bypass procedures. The artery begins at the outer border of the first rib and becomes the brachial artery at the lower border of the teres major muscle.

- The axillary artery is exposed through a lateral infraclavicular incision. The pectoralis major muscle (fig. b) is split between its sternal and clavicular heads.

- The clavipectoral fascia is divided (fig. b). This fascia lies beneath the pectoral fascia and extends vertically from the clavicle to the axillary fascia (fig. b). The pectoralis minor muscle is then identified and retracted laterally to expose the axillary vein (Figs. a and b).

- The axillary vein is retracted inferiorly to expose the axillary artery with the acromiothoracic and superior thoracic arteries (branches of the axillary artery which may be damaged during mobilisation) (fig. a).

- Posterior to the axillary artery lie the lateral, posterior and medial cords of the brachial plexus (fig. b).

Exposure of the Brachial Artery

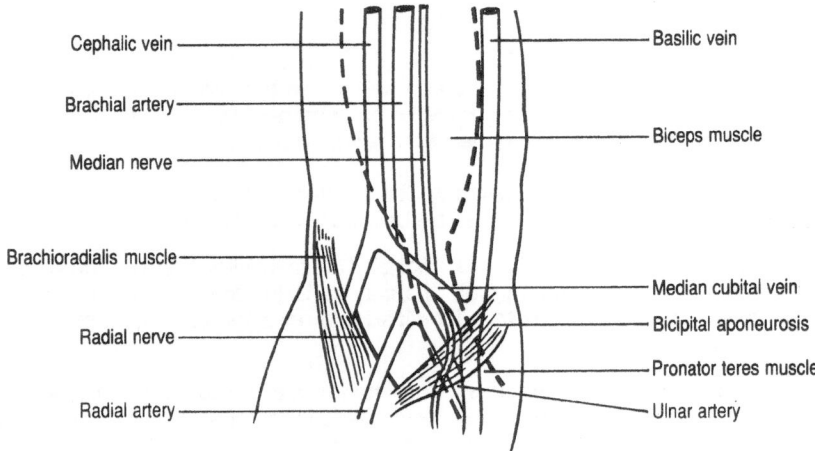

Cephalic vein

Brachial artery

Median nerve

Brachioradialis muscle

Radial nerve

Radial artery

Basilic vein

Biceps muscle

Median cubital vein

Bicipital aponeurosis

Pronator teres muscle

Ulnar artery

FIG. A *Anterior approach to the brachial artery; (– – –) denotes approximate position of the biceps muscle.*

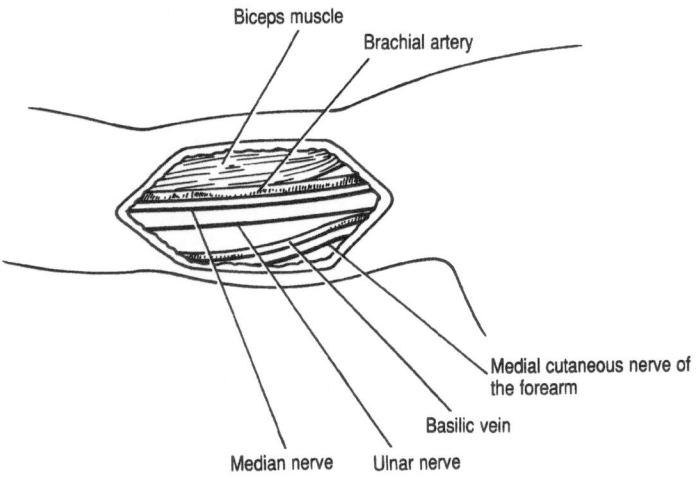

Biceps muscle

Brachial artery

Medial cutaneous nerve of the forearm

Basilic vein

Median nerve

Ulnar nerve

FIG. B *Medial approach to the brachial artery.*

The brachial artery may have to be exposed in order to dislodge an embolus or for exploration after trauma.

Ante-cubital Fossa (Anterior) Approach

- The anterior approach is useful when it is deemed necessary to embolectomise the radial and ulnar arteries separately; a sigmoid-shaped incision can be made. However, the brachial artery may bifurcate high in the arm.

- The distal end of the brachial artery lies in the ante-cubital fossa, a triangular depression lying anterior to the elbow joint. The fossa is bordered by the brachioradialis muscle (laterally), pronator teres muscle (medially) and an imaginary line connecting the two humeral condyles (fig. a).

- By dividing the bicipital aponeurosis the brachial artery is exposed with the median cubital vein crossing it obliquely (fig. a).

- The median nerve lies medial to the brachial artery and the radial nerve lies inferior to the brachioradialis muscle (fig. a).

Medial Approach

- The incision is made in the line of the artery along the medial edge of the biceps muscle. The basilic vein and the medial cutaneous nerve of the forearm are superficial to the deep fascia at this level (fig. b).

- The deep fascia is divided and the inner fibres of the biceps muscle are retracted upwards. The brachial artery should then be found lying on the triceps muscle, with the median nerve anterior to it (fig. b).

- Lying with the brachial artery will be two venae comitantes.

Carotid Endarterectomy

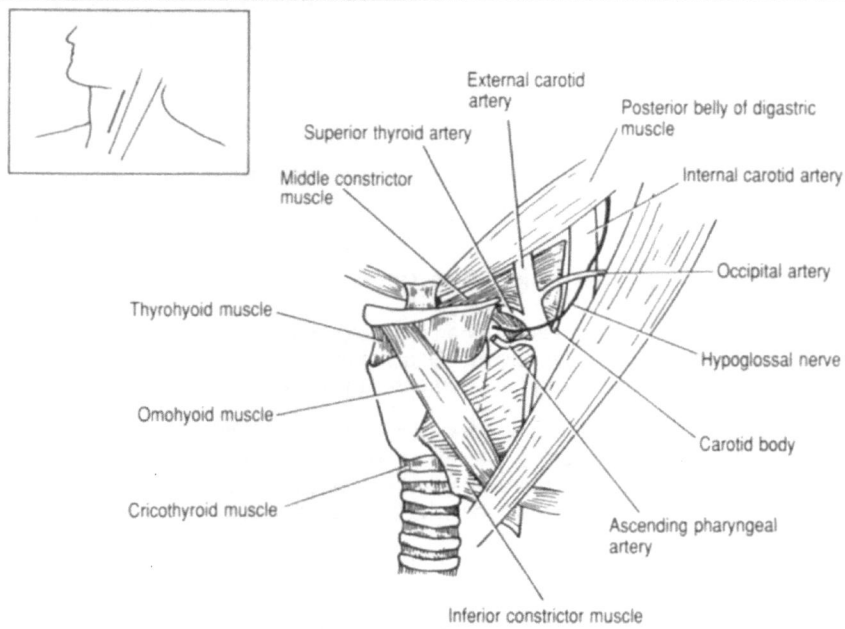

FIG. A *The carotid triangle containing the common carotid artery bifurcation.*

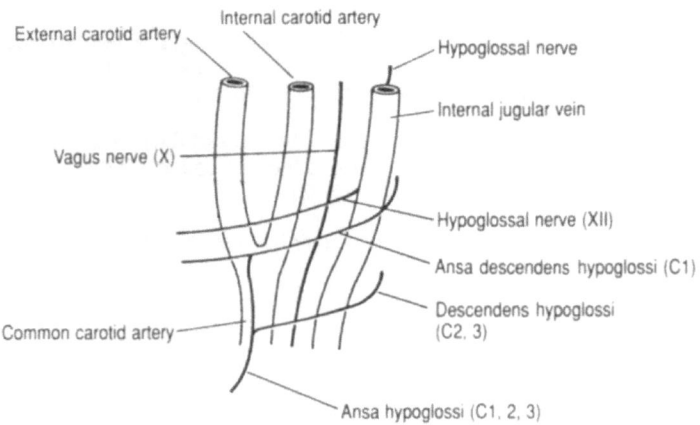

FIG. B *The carotid bifurcation and related nerves.*

Carotid Endarterectomy

The common carotid artery divides into its internal and external branches at the level of the upper border of the thyroid cartilage (lower border of C3). The external carotid artery lies anteriorly, giving off the occipital artery which crosses both the internal carotid artery and the hypoglossal nerve (fig. a). The common carotid bifurcation can be identified in the carotid triangle, which is bounded superiorly by the posterior belly of the digastric muscle, medially by the omohyoid muscle and laterally by sternomastoid muscles. The internal jugular vein is lateral to the common carotid artery within the carotid sheath (fig. b).

- The surgical approach to the internal carotid artery is via an incision along the anterior border of the sternomastoid muscle. This is similar to the approach for excision of a pharyngeal pouch and branchial fistula (see pp. 14 and 16).

- The carotid body, situated at the bifurcation of the common carotid artery, is injected by some surgeons with local anaesthetic to prevent hypotension from developing during mobilisation of the internal carotid artery (fig. a).

- During mobilisation of the common carotid artery the superior thyroid, ascending pharyngeal and occipital arteries can be identified and preserved (fig. a).

- The internal and external carotid arteries are crossed superficially by the hypoglossal and ansa descendens hypoglossi (C1) nerves; the latter travels to supply the geniohyoid and thyrohyoid muscles (fig. b).

- The descendens hypoglossi (C2, 3) travels around the internal jugular vein and joins a branch of the ansa descendens hypoglossi to form the ansa cervicalis, which is embedded in the anterior wall of the carotid sheath and supplies the sternohyoid, sternothyroid and omohyoid muscles (strap muscles) (fig. b).

Lumbar Sympathectomy

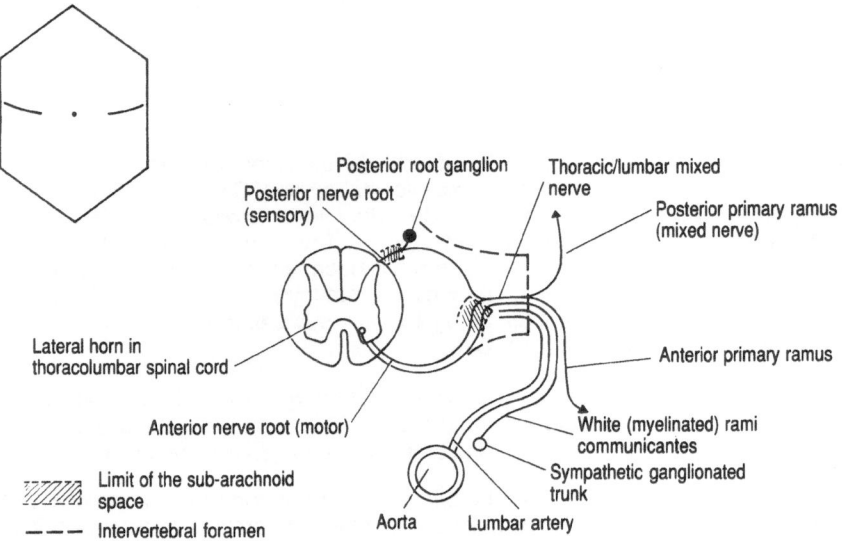

FIG. A *Transverse section (left) of the spinal cord, aorta and spinal nerve.*

Posterior root ganglion

Thoracic/lumbar mixed nerve

Posterior nerve root (sensory)

Posterior primary ramus (mixed nerve)

Lateral horn in thoracolumbar spinal cord

Anterior primary ramus

Anterior nerve root (motor)

White (myelinated) rami communicantes

Sympathetic ganglionated trunk

Limit of the sub-arachnoid space

Intervertebral foramen

Aorta   Lumbar artery

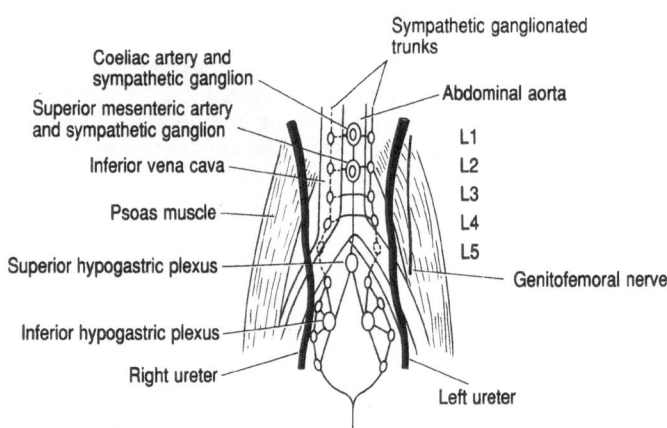

FIG. B *Relations of the sympathetic ganglionated trunk showing the connections between the sympathetic plexus and ganglia.*

Coeliac artery and sympathetic ganglion

Sympathetic ganglionated trunks

Superior mesenteric artery and sympathetic ganglion

Abdominal aorta

Inferior vena cava

L1
L2
L3
L4
L5

Psoas muscle

Superior hypogastric plexus

Genitofemoral nerve

Inferior hypogastric plexus

Right ureter

Left ureter

Lumbar Sympathectomy

The autonomic sympathetic innervation of the lower limb arises in the spinal cord from segments T10–L2. Autonomic fibres pass out of the intervertebral foramina in mixed lumbar nerves. They then travel with the anterior primary rami, eventually branching out via the white rami communicantes to connect with the lumbar sympathetic ganglionated trunk (fig. a). Complete sympathectomy of the calf and foot can be achieved by excising the L2 and L3 lumbar ganglia. The lumbar sympathetic chain can be excised by an anterolateral extraperitoneal approach, or by an anterior transperitoneal approach (not described) simultaneously performed with aorto-iliac bypass surgery.

Anterolateral Extraperitoneal Approach

- An oblique incision is made from the tip of the 12th rib extending into the iliac fossa midway between the umbilicus and the anterior superior iliac spine. A gridiron muscle-splitting approach is made through the anterior abdominal wall muscles into the extraperitoneal space where the peritoneum can be swept anteriorly.

- The ureter will lie anteriorly due to its attachment to the parietal peritoneum, but must be positively identified to prevent trauma (fig. b).

- The genitofemoral nerve lies posteriorly on the iliopsoas muscle (fig. b) and should not be mistaken for the sympathetic ganglionated trunk.

- The sympathetic trunk lies medial to the psoas muscle over the transverse processes of the lumbar vertebrae. On the left side the chain lies adjacent and lateral to the aorta; on the right it lies underneath the lateral edge of the inferior vena cava (fig. b). Identification is achieved by defining the ganglia, which form discrete swellings along the length of the chain.

- Care must be taken to avoid haemorrhage from lumbar arteries and veins (fig. a), which cross horizontally and lie posteriorly to the sympathetic ganglionated trunk.

Above Knee Amputation

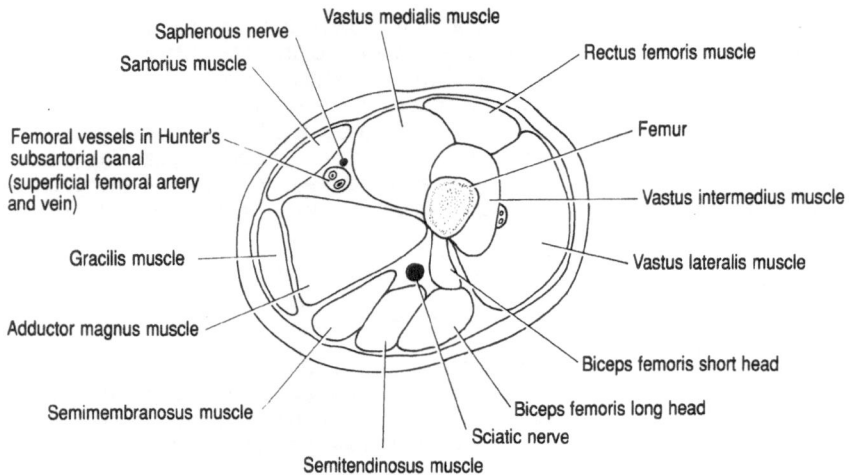

FIG. A   *Cross section through the thigh.*

- Equal anterior and posterior skin flaps are fashioned, deepening the incisions through fat and deep fascia.

- Having made the appropriate incision and deepened it through the skin, fat and deep fascia (fig. a), sartorius and vastus medialis are identified. The superficial femoral artery and vein lie beneath these muscles with the saphenous nerve (fig. a).

- The sartorius muscle, which runs obliquely across the thigh from its lateral origin at the anterior superior iliac spine to its medial insertion to the tibia, should be identified. The vascular bundle containing the superficial femoral artery and vein lies beneath this muscle in Hunter's subsartorial canal (fig. a).

- The quadriceps, hamstrings and the medial muscle groups (sartorius, gracilis and adductor magnus muscles) have to be transected in order to complete the amputation (fig. a)

- The sciatic nerve lies in the posterior compartment of the thigh between the hamstring muscles posterolaterally and adductor magnus medially (fig. a). The nerve should be sectioned at as high a level as possible.

- Using a myoplastic technique to fashion the stump the iliotibial tract is sewn to the adductor magnus and the hamstring group to the quadriceps group of muscles.

Below Knee Amputation

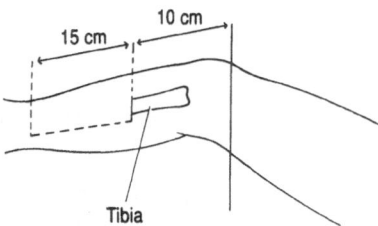

FIG. A *Skin flaps for below knee amputation.*

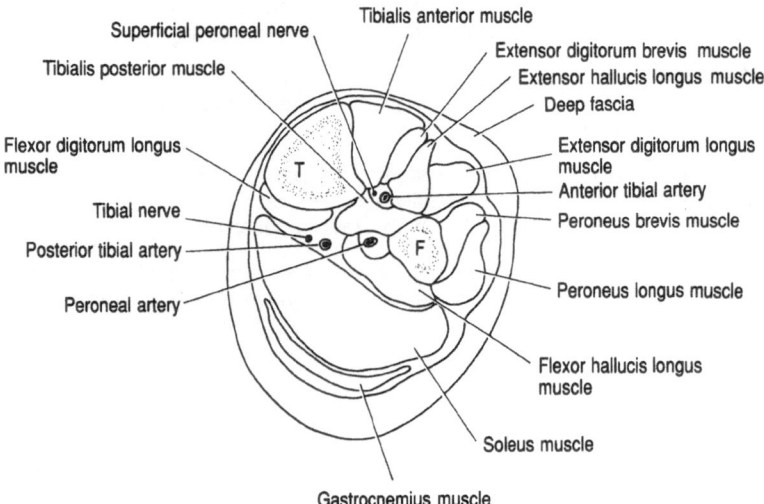

FIG. B *Cross section through the calf. F, fibula; T, tibia.*

Below knee amputation can be performed using equal anterior and posterior flaps. However, most surgeons now opt for a technique with a long posterior flap or "skew" flaps to achieve better healing and a more robust stump. The anatomical features in a long posterior flap amputation are described.

- Skin flaps are mapped out as shown in fig. a.

- The muscles of the extensor compartment (tibialis anterior, extensor digitorum longus and peroneus longus) are divided at the level of the upper incision. Once the muscles have been divided the superficial peroneal and tibial nerves can be identified and sectioned (fig. b). If patent, the anterior tibial artery will require ligation and/or transfixation.

- The tibia can now be divided below the knee joint. The fibula is exposed and divided below the knee joint.

- The tibialis anterior muscle in the extensor compartment of the leg is divided with the deep peroneal nerve (fig. b).

- In order to divide the fibula it must be anterolaterally cleared of the peroneus longus and brevis muscles (fig. b). Between these muscles lies the superficial peroneal nerve.

- After division of the tibia and fibula a tissue plane can be entered between the tibialis posterior and the soleus and gastrocnemius muscles. The posterior tibial nerve and posterior tibial artery are located within this plane and divided (fig. c). The peroneal artery is lateral to the posterior tibial neurovascular bundle between the interosseous membrane and the flexor hallucis longus muscle (fig. c).

- The bulky muscle flap of soleus and gastrocnemius usually has to be reduced by thinning to achieve the correct contour for the stump. The wound is closed by suturing the deep fascia over the gastrocnemius muscle to the anterior tibial periosteum.

Varicose Vein Surgery

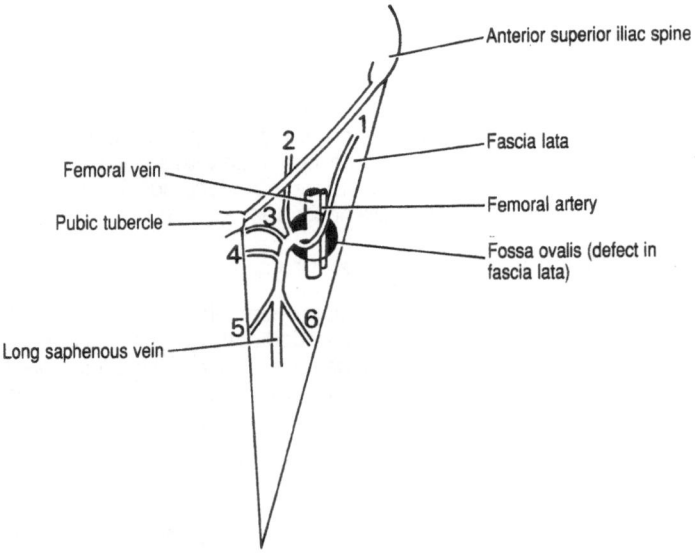

FIG. A *Femoral triangle showing entrance of the long saphenous vein through the fossa ovalis into the femoral vein. Tributaries of the long saphenous vein: 1, superficial circumflex iliac; 2, superficial epigastric; 3, superficial external pudendal; 4, deep external pudendal; 5, medial femoral; 6, lateral femoral.*

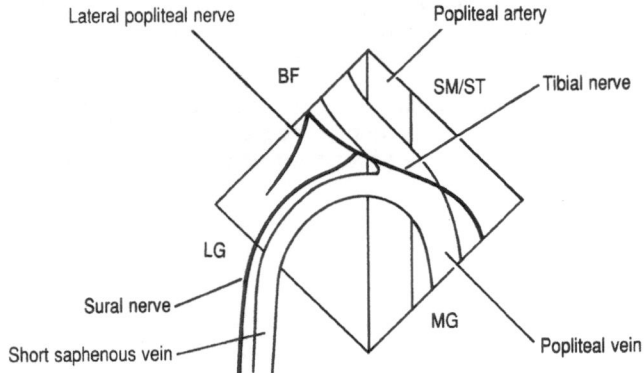

FIG. B *The saphenopopliteal junction. BF, biceps femoris; SM/ST, semimembranosus/semitendinosus; MG, medial head of gastrocnemius; LG, lateral head of gastrocnemius.*

In the presence of established reflux the main aim of varicose vein surgery is to ligate the long saphenous vein at the saphenofemoral junction. If short saphenous vein reflux is demonstrated this vein should be ligated at its junction with the popliteal vein behind the knee in the popliteal fossa.

The Saphenofemoral Junction

- The long saphenous vein courses up the leg from a point anterior to the medial malleolus along the medial aspect of the calf, knee and thigh to join the femoral vein via a defect in the fascia lata: the fossa ovalis (fig. a).

- In a high ligation procedure the tributaries of the long saphenous vein close to the saphenofemoral junction are divided (fig. a).

- The proximal end of the long saphenous vein should be dissected fully so that the junction can be clearly identified. This allows accurate placement of a ligature and avoids potential damage to the femoral vein.

- Some surgeons strip the long saphenous vein to the knee and others to the ankle. However, stripping the vein to the ankle risks damage to the saphenous nerve. It has also been suggested that the distal portion of the vein below the knee should be retained for possible use in coronary artery bypass grafting.

Saphenopopliteal Junction

- The short saphenous vein commences behind the lateral malleolus and runs up the posterior aspect of the leg penetrating the deep fascia over the popliteal fossa to join the popliteal vein (fig. b).

- The short saphenous vein is intimately related to the sural nerve in the popliteal fossa (fig. b).

- The site of the saphenopopliteal junction is variable and may be difficult to identify due to fat and lymphatic tissue in the popliteal fossa. Precise anatomical localisation can be obtained pre-operatively by venography or Duplex Doppler scanning.

The superficial and deep venous systems are connected in the thigh and calf by perforating veins. In the presence of perforator incompetence sub-fascial ligation of these veins can be performed (Cocketts' procedure).

IV. Miscellaneous

Surgical Exposure of the Kidney

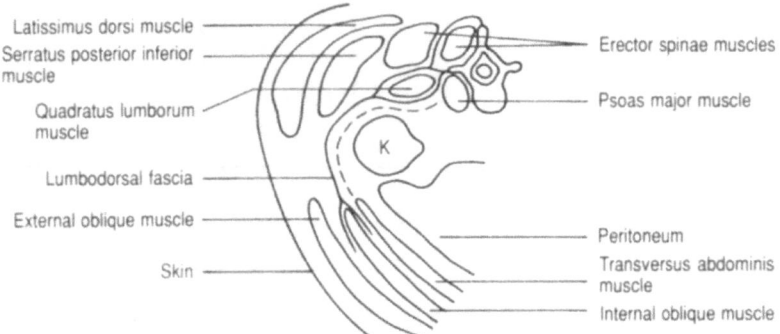

Latissimus dorsi muscle

Serratus posterior inferior muscle

Quadratus lumborum muscle

Lumbodorsal fascia

External oblique muscle

Skin

Erector spinae muscles

Psoas major muscle

K

Peritoneum

Transversus abdominis muscle

Internal oblique muscle

FIG. A   *Transverse section through the loin demonstrating the subcostal approach to the kidney (K). The dashed line indicates the course of the subcostal nerve.*

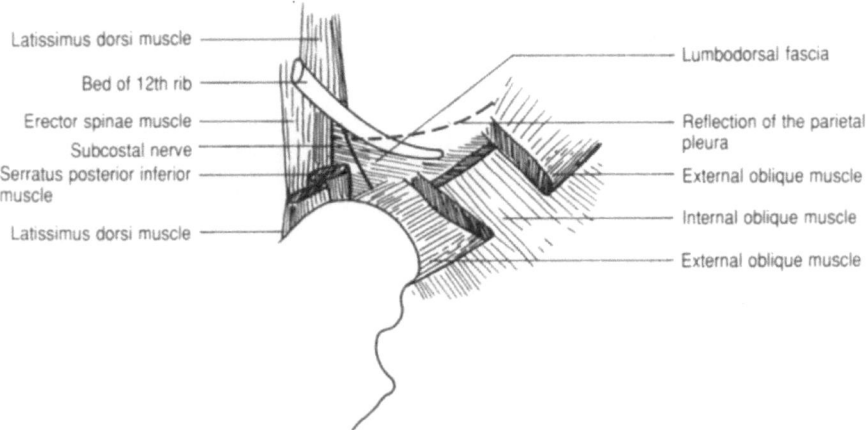

Latissimus dorsi muscle

Bed of 12th rib

Erector spinae muscle

Subcostal nerve

Serratus posterior inferior muscle

Latissimus dorsi muscle

Lumbodorsal fascia

Reflection of the parietal pleura

External oblique muscle

Internal oblique muscle

External oblique muscle

FIG. B   *Lateral aspect of the loin.*

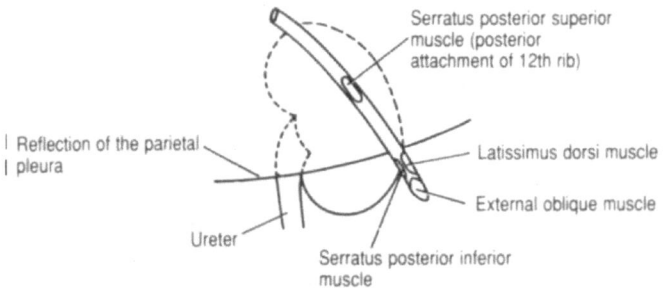

Serratus posterior superior muscle (posterior attachment of 12th rib)

Reflection of the parietal pleura

Latissimus dorsi muscle

External oblique muscle

Ureter

Serratus posterior inferior muscle

FIG. C   *Posterior aspect of the loin (right) to demonstrate the relationship of the kidney to the 12th rib and pleural reflection.*

The standard surgical approach to the kidney is through the loin using a subcostal or transcostal route. Surgery for renal tumours may require either anterior abdominal exploration or loin and abdominal incisions if a total nephro-ureterectomy is being performed. The commonly used subcostal and transcostal approaches to the kidney are described.

Subcostal Approach

- The incision extends from the angle of the 12th rib and the anterior border of the erector spinae muscles, and passes forwards 1 cm below and parallel to the 12th rib to a point 2 cm above the anterior superior iliac spine.

- The fibres of the external oblique muscle run in the line of the incision anteriorly with latissimus dorsi, forming the superficial muscle layer at the posterior end of the wound (fig. a).

- The serratus posterior inferior muscle lies deep to latissimus dorsi. Division of serratus posterior inferior exposes the lateral edge of the erector spinae muscle and the lumbodorsal fascia. The subcostal nerve lying deep to the lumbodorsal fascia should be preserved (fig. b).

- Division of the internal oblique muscle and the lumbodorsal fascia exposes the perinephric space (fig. a). Anteriorly the peritoneum has to be carefully separated from the transversus abdominis muscle to prevent tearing of the peritoneum and to aid access to the kidney.

Transcostal Approach

- The incision is made along the line of the 12th rib, dividing the serratus posterior inferior and latissimus dorsi muscles.

- The 12th rib is resected after incising the periosteum and elevating it from the upper surface of the rib, taking care not to damage the pleura (fig. c).

- The lumbodorsal fascia is divided to gain entry into the perinephric space (figs. a and b).

Approaches to the Ureter

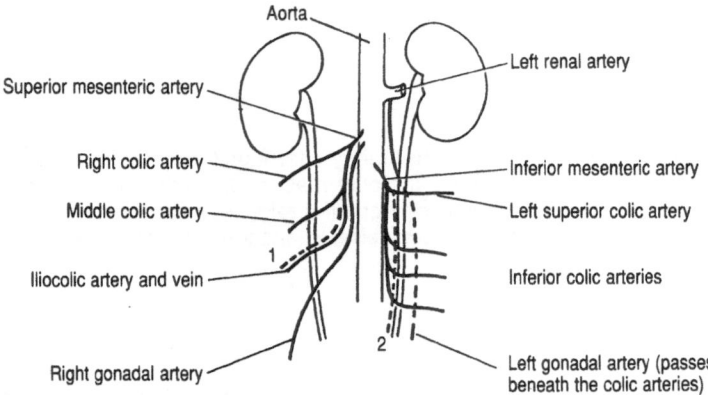

FIG. A *Main anterior vascular relations of the ureter. 1, superior mesenteric vein; 2, inferior mesenteric vein.*

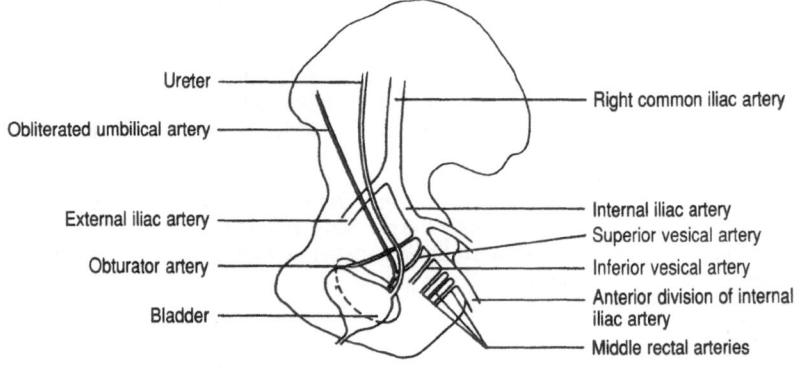

FIG. B *Lateral relations of the ureter.*

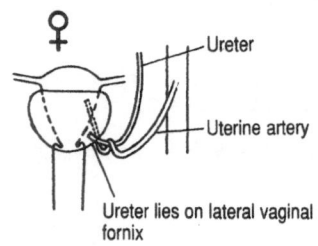

Ureter is crossed superiorly by the uterine artery:

FIG. C *Pelvic relations of the ureter in the female (posterior view).*

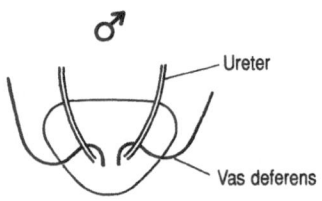

FIG. D *Pelvic relations of the ureter in the male (posterior view, vas deferens crosses ureter anteriorly).*

Lithotripsy and percutaneous surgery have reduced the need for open procedures to extract renal calculi. However, it is still sometimes necessary to expose the ureter to remove an impacted stone or to carry out repair. The approach to the ureter depends upon the site of the stone.

Upper Third

- A subcostal approach can be used as described for exposing the kidney (p. 84). The renal vessels are anterior to the pelvis and ureter.

- Having identified the ureter it should be mobilised so that a sufficient length is available for ureterolithotomy. Extensive mobilisation may damage the ureteric blood supply (fig. a), which is mainly derived from small vessels running with the ureter in the surrounding connective tissue and overlying peritoneum.

Middle Third

- A loin incision is made and the ureter exposed after dividing the external oblique, internal oblique and transversus abdominis muscles (a similar retroperitoneal approach as for lumbar sympathectomy: see p. 74).

- The peritoneum should be gently swept forwards with the hand.

- The ureter is mobilised carefully to avoid bleeding from a gonadal vein (fig. a).

Lower Third

- Pfannenstiel's incision can be used.

- The peritoneum has to be carefully retracted upwards.

- The ureter should be identified as it crosses the common iliac artery and followed down into the pelvis (fig. b).

- The superior vesical vascular pedicle may have to be divided to allow visualisation of the lower end of the ureter. The pedicle can be identified by following the obliterated umbilical artery downwards (fig. b).

- The ureter is crossed superiorly and anteriorly by the uterine artery in the female (fig. c) and by the vas deferens in the male (fig. d).

Simple Mastectomy

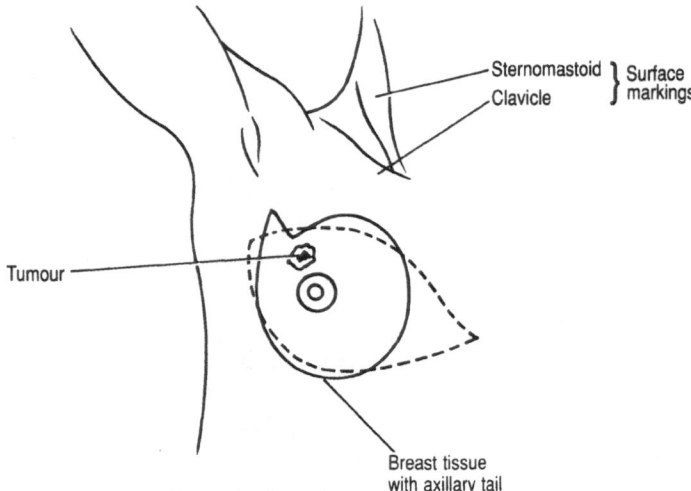

FIG. A *The superior and inferior skin flaps for simple mastectomy.*

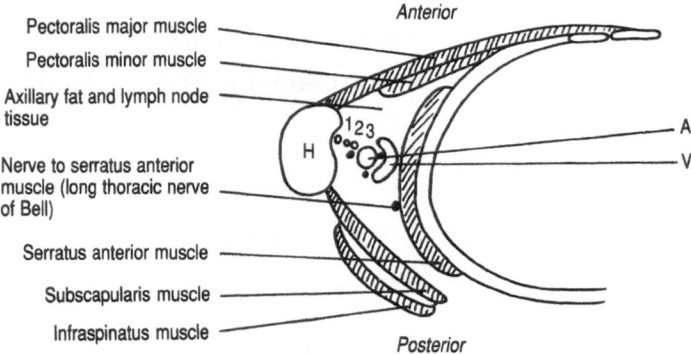

FIG. B *Transverse section through the axilla. 1, long head of biceps tendon; 2, short head of biceps tendon; 3, coracobrachialis tendon; A, axillary artery; V, axillary vein and lateral, medial and posterior cords of the brachial plexus; H, humerus.*

In a standard simple mastectomy operation the breast disc and its axillary tail are excised with an ellipse of skin which includes the nipple. The skin ellipse is usually placed obliquely as shown in fig. a, but in some patients a more cosmetic result may be obtained with flaps that result in a transverse scar.

- The lines of incision should be carefully marked so that the edges of the superior and inferior flaps can be sewn together without undue tension (fig. a).

- A plane is developed between the underside of the skin and the breast tissue. The incisions are deepened to incise the deep fascia overlying the pectoralis major muscle. The fascia is excised in continuity with the specimen.

- Medially care should be taken to achieve haemostasis from branches of the internal mammary artery (a branch of the first part of the subclavian artery).

- Laterally the long thoracic nerve of Bell (the nerve to the serratus anterior muscle should be preserved) (fig. b).

Removal of Axillary Lymph Nodes

Removal of the axillary lymph nodes may form part of a radical (e.g. Patey) or simple mastectomy. Alternatively it may be performed as a separate procedure when a malignant lump has been removed from the breast.

- Care must be taken to avoid damage to the long thoracic nerve of Bell, which lies medially on the serratus anterior muscle. The axillary vein, which crosses the apex of the axilla (fig. b), is at risk if the operation attempts to achieve a complete clearance of the axillary contents (fat and lymph nodes).

- High up in the axilla haemostasis should be performed with ties and not diathermy to avoid the risk of damage to the cords and branches of the brachial plexus (fig. b).

Microdochectomy

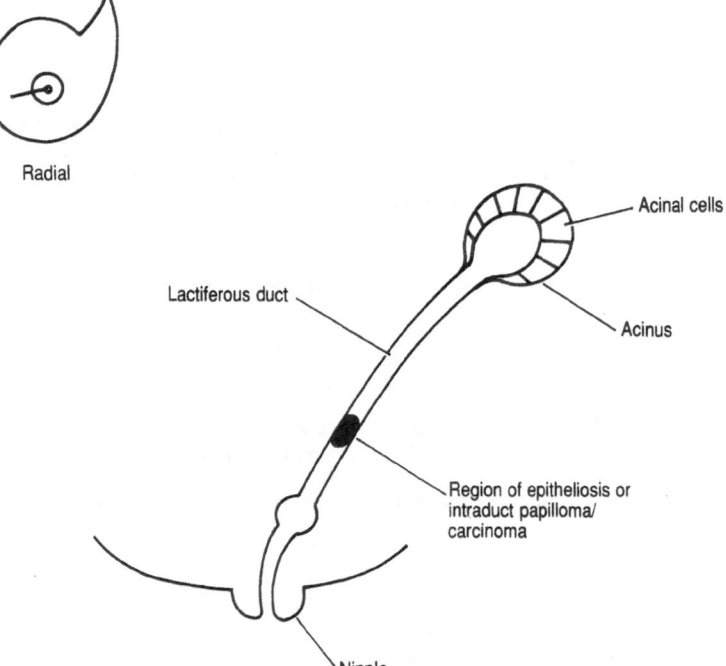

Radial

Acinal cells

Lactiferous duct

Acinus

Region of epitheliosis or
intraduct papilloma/
carcinoma

Nipple

FIG. A   *Basic structure of the breast and the ductal
system excised in microdochectomy.*

Microdochectomy

Microdochectomy is indicated in patients with blood-stained or serous nipple discharge where the origin of the discharge from a single duct orifice can be identified.

- The lactiferous ducts radiate out circumferentially from the breast and when probed care should be taken not to form a false passage (fig. a).

- The whole ductal system on either side of the probe should be excised beyond the areolar region and out into the breast tissue.